Pharmacogenetics

Edited by Islam A. Khalil

Published in London, United Kingdom

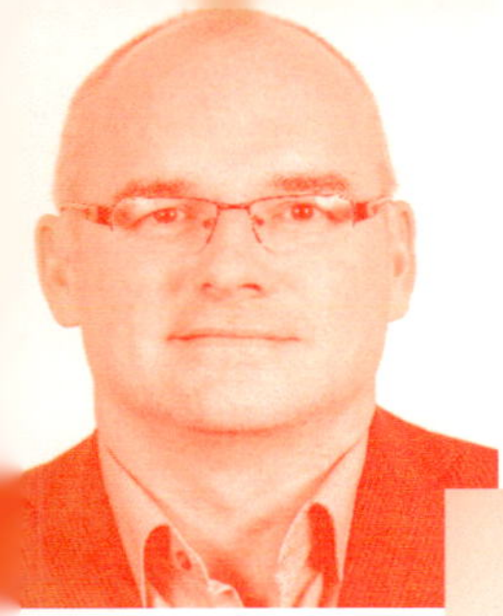
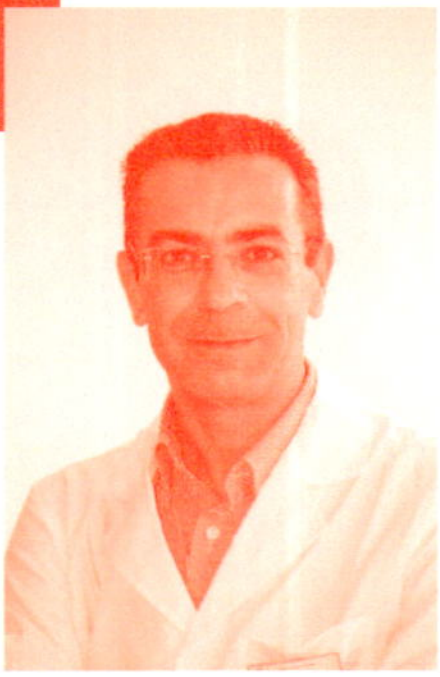
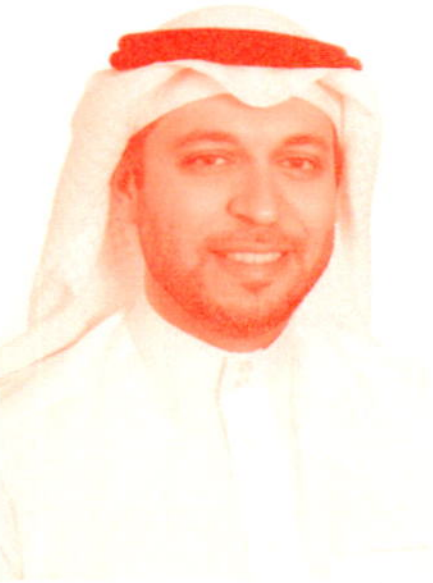
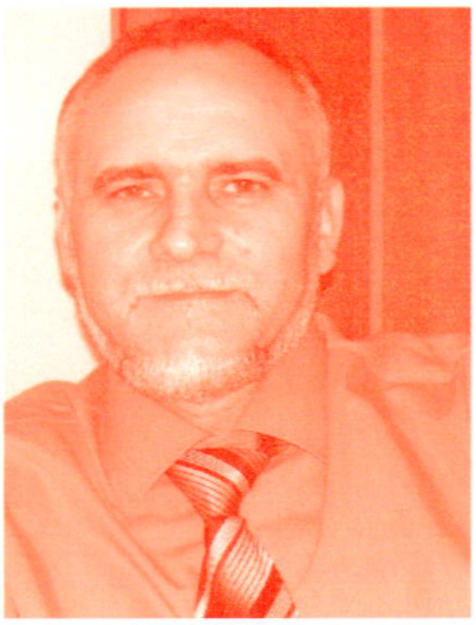
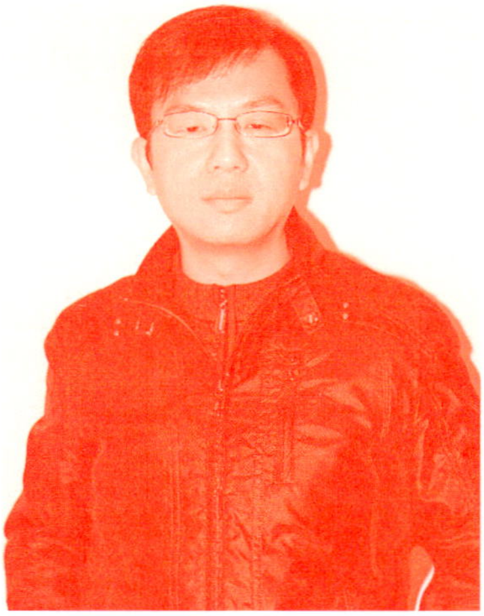
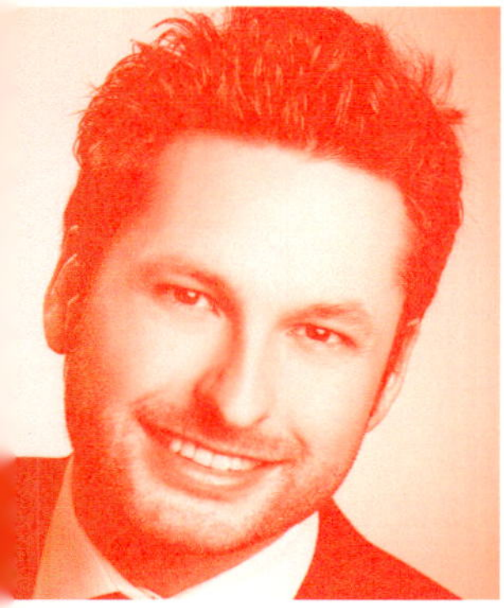
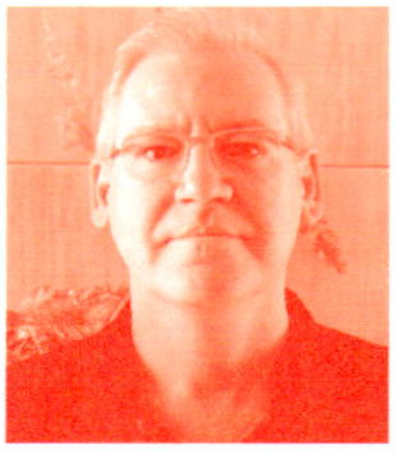

IntechOpen

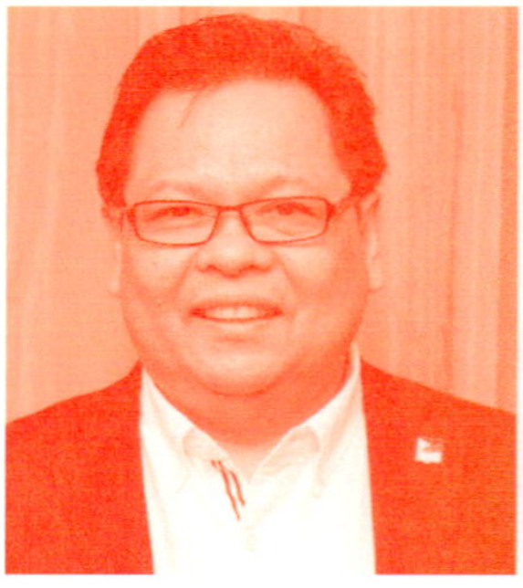
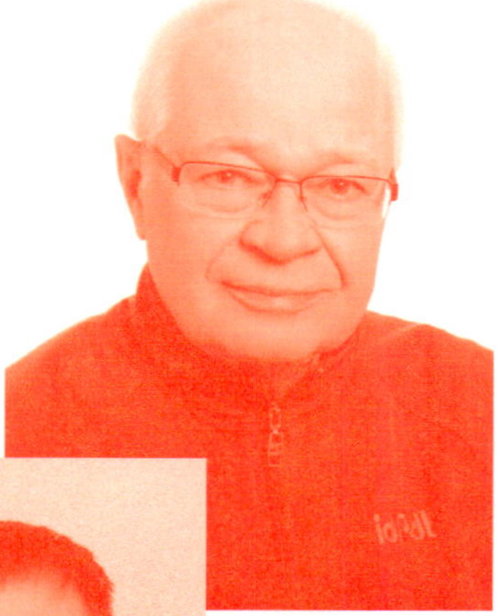
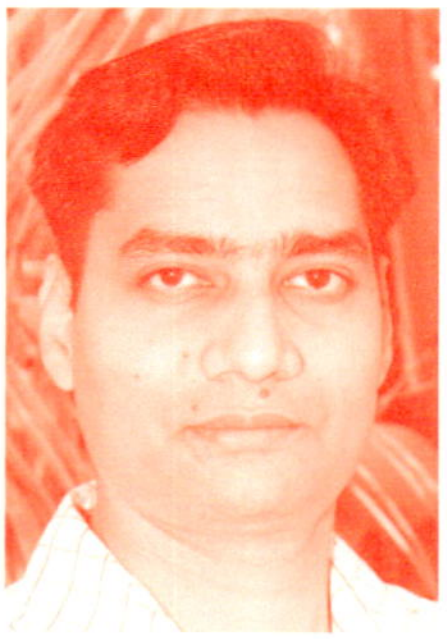
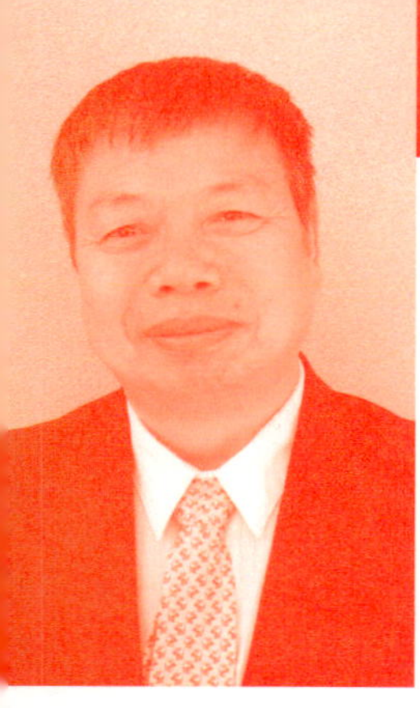
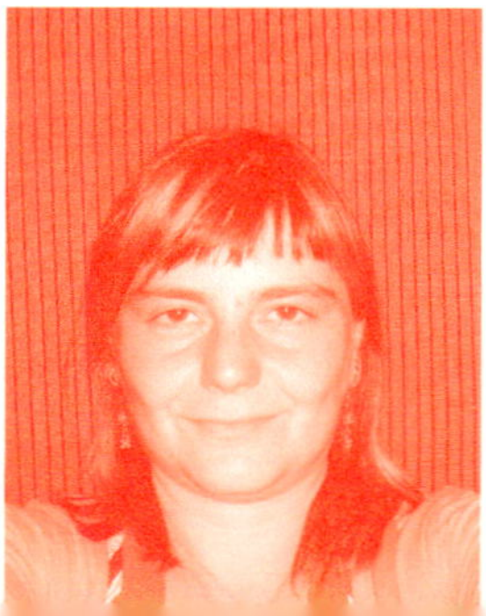
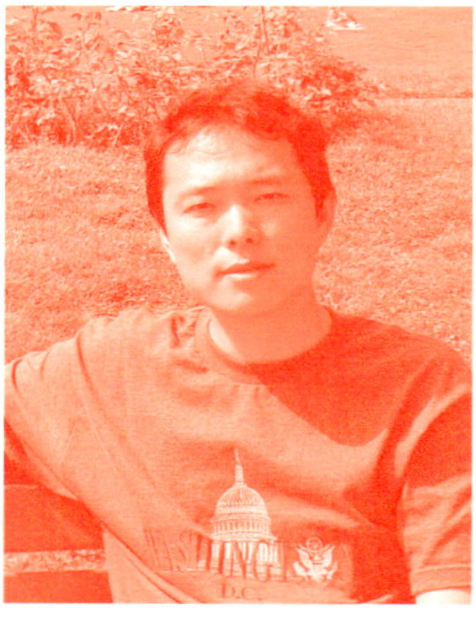

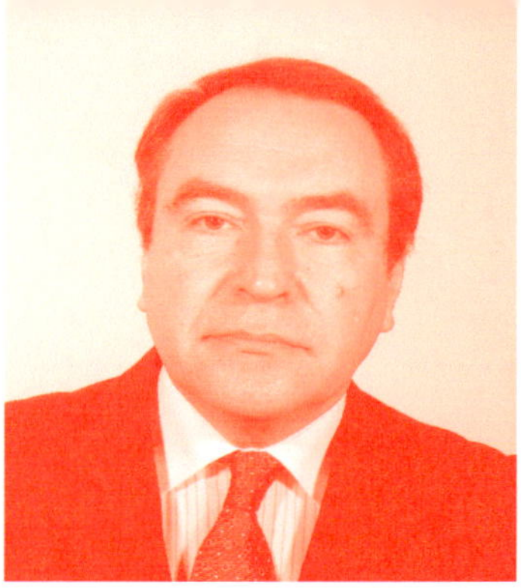
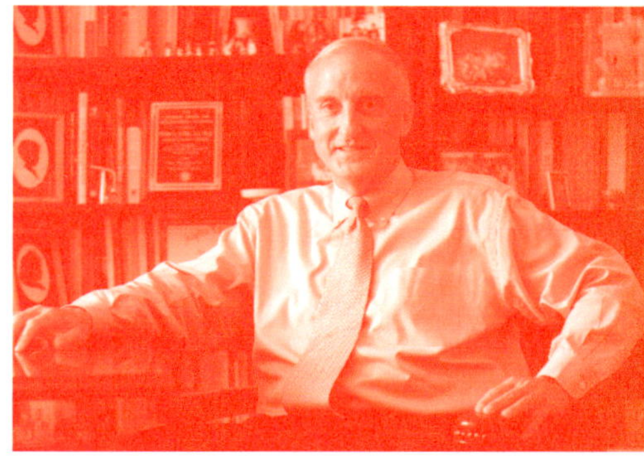
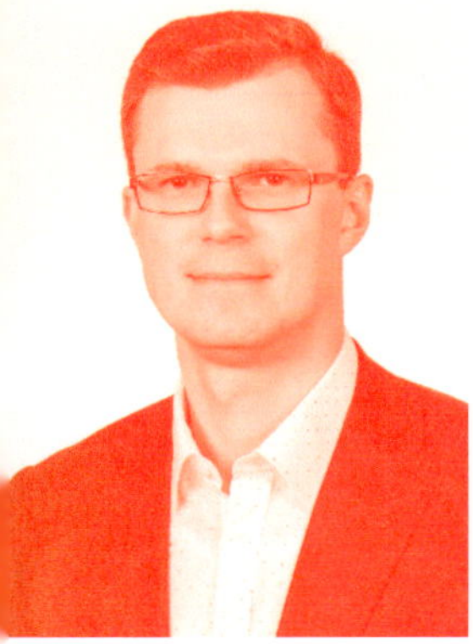
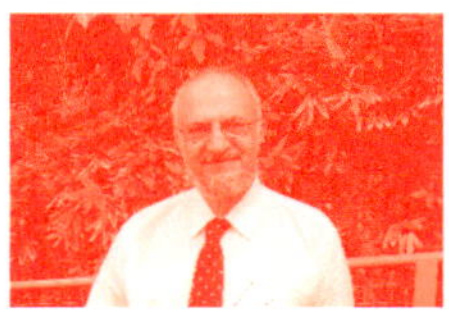
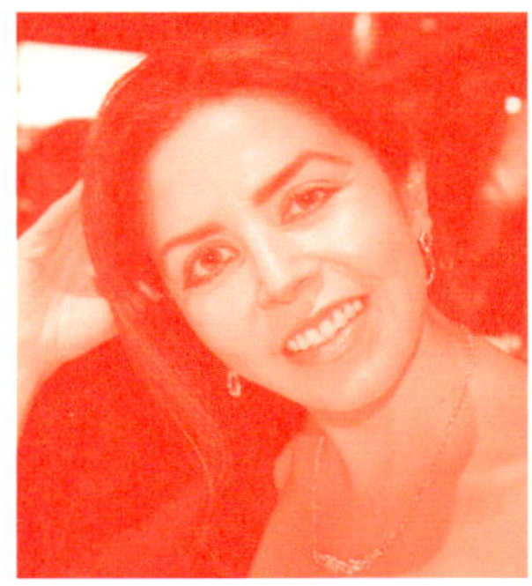

Supporting open minds since 2005

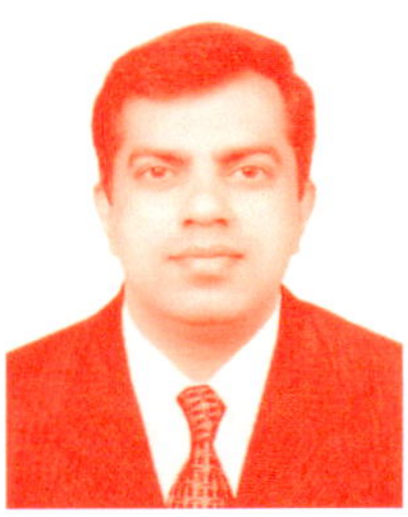
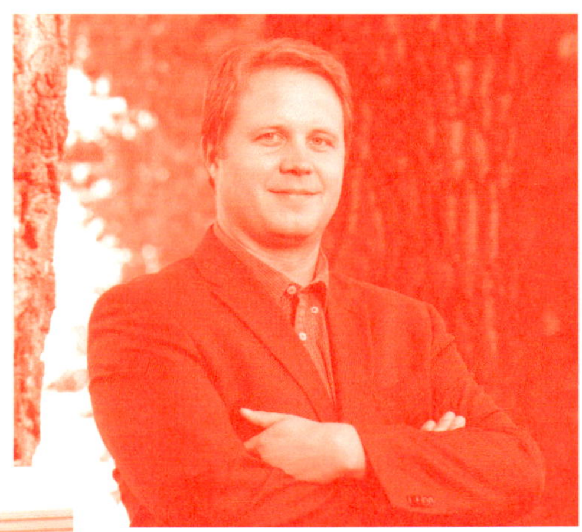
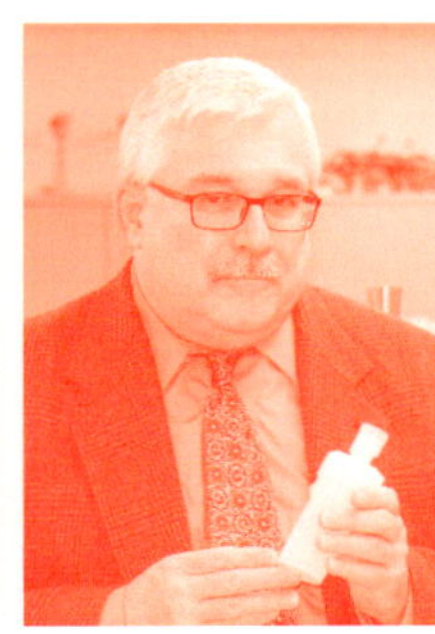
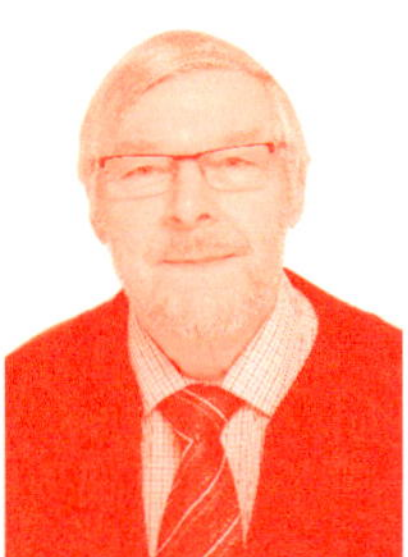
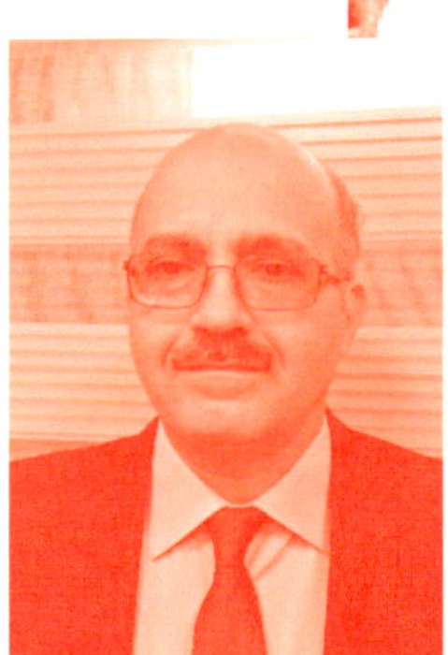
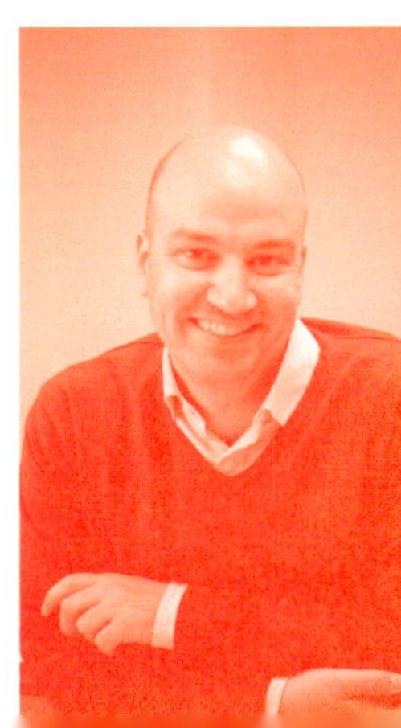
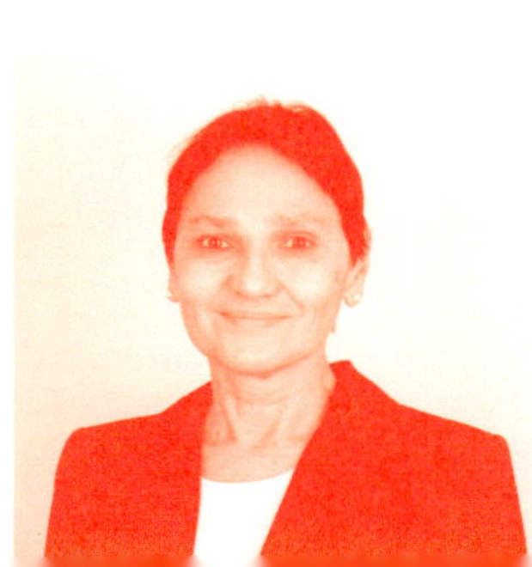

Pharmacogenetics
http://dx.doi.org/10.5772/intechopen.92954
Edited by Islam A. Khalil

Contributors
Dmitriy A. Anatolyevich Kuznetsov, Valentin V. Vladimirovich Fursov, Alexander A. Bukhvostov, Ilia V. Fursov, Aleksander G. Majouga, Manash Paul, Keshav Moharir, Munindra Ruwali, Sanjiv Singh, Punita Aggarwal, Jose Antonio DIniz Oliveira, Abdulmohsen Alrohaimi, Kholoud Saeed Aldmasi, Nada Hussain Alruwais, Bader Alrohaimi, ruchi chawla, Varsha Rani, Mohini Mishra, Krishan Kumar, Natalia A Shnayder, Marina Petrova, Elena Bochanova, Olga Zimnitskaya, Alina Savinova, Regina Nasyrova, Elena Pozhilenkova, Debasish Mukhopadhyay, Priyanka Sengupta, Molungoa Sello, Islam A. Khalil

First published in London, United Kingdom, 2021 by IntechOpen
IntechOpen is the global imprint of INTECHOPEN LIMITED, registered in England and Wales, registration number: 11086078, 5 Princes Gate Court, London, SW7 2QJ, United Kingdom
Printed in Croatia

British Library Cataloguing-in-Publication Data
A catalogue record for this book is available from the British Library

Additional hard and PDF ccpies can be obtained from orders@intechopen.com

Pharmacogenetics
Edited by Islam A. Khalil
p. cm.
Print ISBN 978-1-83969-217-8
Online ISBN 978-1-83969-218-5
eBook (PDF) ISBN 978-1-83969-219-2

For EU product safety concerns:
IN TECH d.o.o., Prolaz Marije Krucifikse Kozulić 3, 51000 Rijeka, Croatia, info@intechopen.com or visit our website at intechopen.com.

Meet the editor

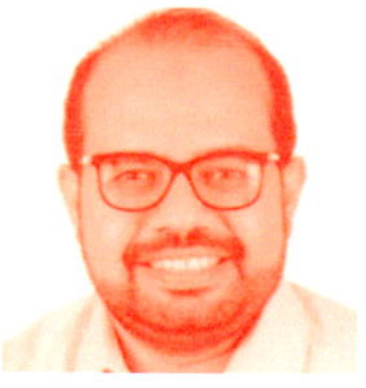

Islam A. Khalil received a BSc in Pharmaceutical Sciences from Misr University for Science and Technology, Egypt, in 2003, and an MSc and Ph.D. in Pharmaceutics from the Faculty of Pharmacy, Cairo University, Egypt, in 2009 and 2013, respectively. Currently, Dr. Khalil is Associate Professor of Pharmaceutics at the College of Pharmacy and Drug Manufacturing, Misr University for Science and Technology, Egypt. He worked previously as a postdoctoral research fellow in an American university in Cairo (Egypt), Zewail City for Science and Technology (Egypt), Brigham and Women's Hospital - Harvard Medical School (USA), and Northeastern University (USA). His research activities focus on designing, developing, and evaluating nanomedicines for various biomedical applications, especially therapeutics and tissue regeneration. He also has considerable industrial research and development experiences to his credit. He received several awards including Best Applied Pharmaceutical Research in 2018 from the Arab Company for Drug Industries and Medical Appliances (ACDIMA) and the State Encouragement Award in Medical Sciences in 2020.

Contents

Preface

Pharmacogenetics is the study of the effects of individual genetics on drug responses. Many studies have investigated the impact of gene variation on the pharmacokinetics and pharmacodynamics of different drugs. This book provides an overview of the current state of the pharmacological genetic aspects of these treatments. It also discusses drugs with genetic information to support product labeling, clinical guidelines, and significant mechanical effects. At this point, clinically relevant genetic variation in drug-metabolizing enzymes may inform the dosage of certain drugs metabolized in the liver. In addition, genetic variation in immune genes can be tested to assess the risk of serious hypersensitivity reactions to certain drugs.

Pharmacogenetic studies mainly focus on the difference in pharmacokinetic parameters after drug administration. It involves clinical investigation of different genes and the effect on biotransformation of drugs to metabolites, for example, tricyclic antidepressants are metabolized at different rates in different populations. Most drugs used to treat neurological and psychiatric diseases are metabolized by the liver. Many genes encoding phase I (oxidation) and phase II (combined) drug-metabolizing enzymes contain genetic polymorphisms that are known to affect their metabolic activity. In addition, the transport proteins expressed in the liver and the function of the blood-brain barrier change the distribution of certain drugs, thereby changing the pharmacokinetic properties. Genetic polymorphisms occurring in drug receptors or other biological targets are thought to be responsible for some of the observed variances in response and tolerance to treatment. For neurological and psychiatric conditions, this may include variations affecting the expression of the target receptor, the structure of the receptor, the arrangement of substances, and neurotransmitters and second messenger pathways. Contrary to the preceding discussion on the pharmacological genetics of drug metabolism, very few drugs currently have genetic markers relevant to pharmacodynamics that are included in product labels or clinical guidelines. Current examples include individuals with immune system genes associated with hypersensitivity risk as well as gene variants associated with inborn errors of metabolism. Although rare, these are clinically important risk factors associated with life-threatening outcomes from some antiepileptic drugs. In addition, numerous studies have been performed to identify and characterize genetic variants related to pharmacodynamics. This book highlights some examples of the impact of pharmacogenetics on different diseases and the use of in silico model for deep understanding.

Islam A. Khalil
Pharmaceutics Department,
College of Pharmacy,
Misr University for Science and Technology,
Giza, Egypt

Section 1

Introduction

Chapter 1

Introductory Chapter: Pharmacogenetics

Islam A. Khalil

1. Introduction

Pharmacogenetics is the study of how individual genetics affect drug responses. Many studies investigated the impact of gene variation on the pharmacokinetic and pharmacodynamic of different drugs. This chapter gives an overview of the current state of the pharmacological genetic aspects of these treatments. Drugs with genetic information to support product labeling, clinical guidelines, or significant mechanical effects are discussed. At this point, clinically relevant genetic variation in drug-metabolizing enzymes may reveal the dosage of certain drugs metabolized in the liver. In addition, genetic variation in immune genes can be tested to assess the risk of serious hypersensitivity reactions to certain drugs.

2. Pharmacogenetics and pharmacokinetics

Pharmacogenetic studies mainly focus on the difference in pharmacokinetic parameters after drug administration. These involve clinical investigation of different genes and their effect on biotransformation of drugs to metabolites; for example, tricyclic antidepressants were metabolized in different rates in different populations [1]. Most drugs used to treat neurological and psychiatric diseases are metabolized by the liver. Many genes encoding phase 1 (oxidation) and phase 2 (combined) drug-metabolizing enzymes contain genetic polymorphisms, which are known to affect their metabolic activity. In addition, the pharmacokinetic profile of certain drugs is highly affected by transport proteins that allow the absorption and distribution. These proteins are mainly expressed in hepatic tissue and in blood–brain barrier. The most common biotransformation enzymes are cytochrome P450 (Phase 1), glucuronidase, and catechol/thiopurine methyltransferase (Phase 2). Furthermore, different neurological drugs are affected by transporters, such as P-glycoprotein.

Genetic variation in drug metabolism can alter the biotransformation of a particular drug and can occur due to a combination of inherited alleles from each parent. The results of the functioning of various combinations of drug-metabolizing enzyme alleles may vary slightly depending on the characteristics of the mutation (e.g., fully inactivated enzyme, altered enzyme expression), but are generally maximal. Five categories are considered clinically relevant: (1) low- or no-enzyme activity, (2) medium-enzyme activity (reduced enzyme activity between normal and poor enzyme), (3) normal-enzyme activity (genetically unchanged enzyme activity), (4) fast-enzyme activity (with less increased enzyme activity compared to normal one), and (5) highly fast-enzyme activity (compared to fast-enzyme activity) [2].

IntechOpen

3. Pharmacogenetics and pharmacodynamics

Genetic polymorphisms occurring in drug receptors or other biological targets are thought to be responsible for some of the observed variances in response and tolerance to treatment. For neurological and psychiatric conditions, this may include variations affecting the expression of the target receptor, the structure of the receptor, the arrangement of substance neurotransmitters, and second messenger pathways. Beside the pharmacokinetic variation due to biotransformation, the pharmacodynamics of few drugs are mainly affected by genetic markers that are mentioned in the clinical guidelines. Three famous examples showing the effect of pharmacodynamic-related genes are hypersensitivity risks related to immunological genes, inborn metabolism variations due to gene variants, and antiepileptic drugs associated with life-threatening consequences. In addition, numerous studies have been performed to identify and characterize genetic variants related to pharmacodynamics. In many cases, these signs may also be related to the risk of an underlying disease or illness. A simple example is the biopharmaceutical aspects of hypersensitivity reactions [3].

4. Personalizing medicine

Personalized medicine was recognized in the early nineteenth century by Sir William Osler who studied the variation in drug responses among individuals. This concept evolved over years genomic information have been incorporated into patient's clinical diagnosis and treatment. The major areas of applied research in this field involve identifying the genetic basis of common diseases, studying how genes and the environment interact to cause human disease, and using pharmacogenetic biomarkers to facilitate more effective drug therapy. Pharmacogenetics has become one of the leading and potentially most actionable areas of the personalized medicine paradigm, as evidenced by the increased availability of clinical pharmacogenetic testing among Clinical Laboratory Improvement Amendments-approved

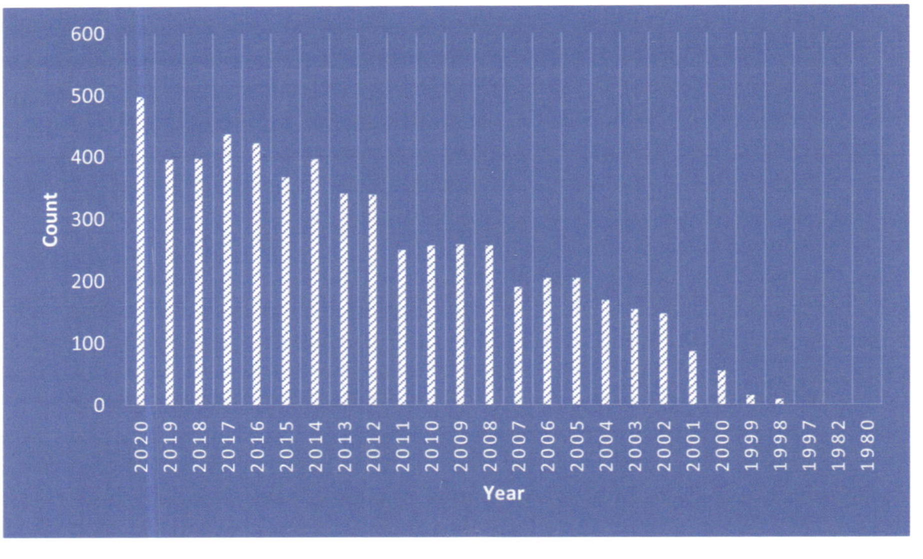

Figure 1.
Number of publications—PubMed citations (http://www.ncbi.nlm.nih.gov/pubmed) by date using the keyword "pharmacogenetics," "pharmacogenomics," or "clinical pharmacogenetics."

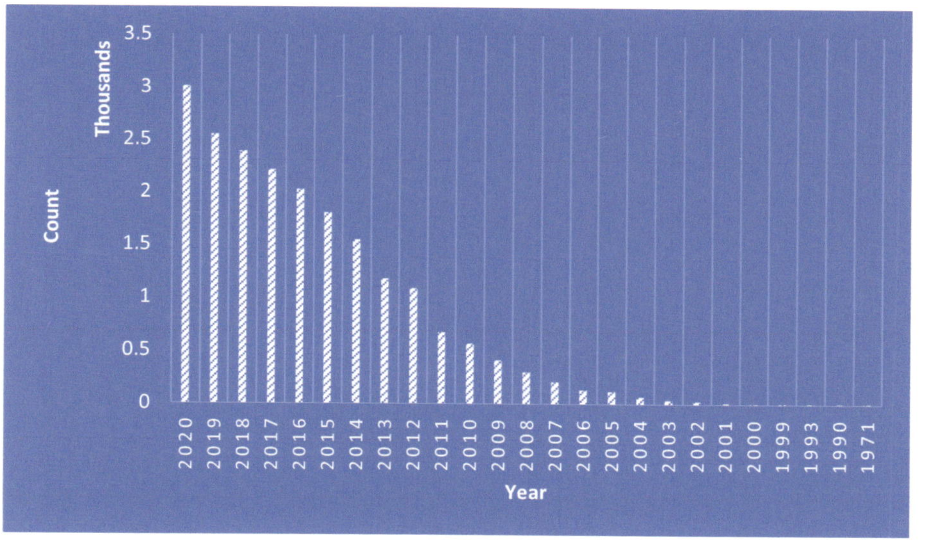

Figure 2.
Number of publications—PubMed citations (http://www.ncbi.nlm.nih.gov/pubmed) by date using the keyword "personalized medicine."

laboratories over the past few years. Moreover, the literature in pharmacogenetic studies over the past decade (**Figure 1**) has proved exponential growth beside FDA acknowledgement. A significant increase was observed starting from 2000 with 55 publications till 2020 with 498 publications. Furthermore, the term personalized medicine (**Figure 1**) was also used from 2000 with 7 publications till 2020 with 3009 publications (**Figure 2**) [4].

In conclusion, pharmacogenetics and personalized medicine showed a rapid growth over years with a great intention to apply the knowledge gained in clinical practice. Important genetic associations have been identified between variant genotypes and drug response phenotypes that encouraged the FDA to revise drug labels to include relevant pharmacological genetic information and recommendations for some certain drugs. However, despite the availability of pharmacological genetic tests from Clinical Laboratory Improvement Amendments-approved laboratories, physician implementation of pharmacological genetic investigation has been unsatisfactory, maybe due to lack of awareness or inadequate professional guidance and limited coverage of testing coverage. Therefore, selected pharmacogenetic examples have been accepted into clinical practice and several others are currently being evaluated in randomized controlled trials.

Author details

Islam A. Khalil
Department of Pharmaceutics, College of Pharmacy and Drug Manufacturing, Misr University of Science and Technology (MUST), Giza, Egypt

*Address all correspondence to: islam.khalil@must.edu.eg

References

[1] Hammer W, Sjöqvist F. Plasma levels of monomethylated tricyclic antidepressants during treatment with imipramine-like compounds. Life Sciences. 1967;**6**(17):1895-1903. DOI: 10.1016/0024-3205(67)90218-4

[2] Caudle KE, Dunnenberger HM, Freimuth RR, Peterson JF, Burlison JD, Whirl-Carrillo M, et al. Standardizing terms for clinical pharmacogenetic test results: Consensus terms from the Clinical Pharmacogenetics Implementation Consortium (CPIC). Genetics in Medicine. 2017;**19**(2): 215-223. DOI: 10.1038/gim.2016.87

[3] Bishop JR. Pharmacogenetics. Handbook of Clinical Neurology. 2018;**147**:59-73. DOI: 10.1016/B978-0-444-63233-3.00006-3

[4] Scott SA. Personalizing medicine with clinical pharmacogenetics. Genetics in Medicine. 2011;**13**(12): 987-995. DOI: 10.1097/gim.0b013e318238b38c

Section 2

Overview on Pharmacogentic

Chapter 2

Integrated Role of Nanotechnology and Pharmacogenetics in Diagnosis and Treatment of Diseases

Ruchi Chawla, Varsha Rani, Mohini Mishra and Krishan Kumar

Abstract

"One size fits all" is an erroneous paradigm in drug delivery, due to side effects/adverse effects and variability observed in drug response. The variability is a result of geneotypic variations (variability in genomic constitution) which is studied in the branch of science called Pharmacogenomics. The variability in drug response is studied by multigene analysis or profiling of whole-genome single nucleotide polymorphism (SNP) and is recorded in terms of the pharmacokinetic (absorption, distribution, metabolism and elimination) and pharmacodynamic (drug-receptor interaction, immune response, etc.) response of the drug. Therefore, a foray into this research area can provide valuable information for designing of drug therapies, identifying disease etiology, therapeutic targets and biomarkers for application in treatment and diagnosis of diseases. Lately, with the integration of pharmacogenomics and nanotechnology, a new facade for the diagnosis and treatment of diseases has opened up, and the prescription pattern of drugs has moved to pharmacotyping (individualized dose and dosage-form adjusted therapy) using nanoplatforms like nanobioconjugates, nanotheranostics, etc.

Keywords: Genome, Personalized, nanotheranostics, Genotyping, Nanomedicines

1. Introduction

By the end of 1950s, pharmacogenetics had become a more established approach for the treatment of diseases. The term 'pharmacogenetics' was coined in the year 1959 by Vogel [1] and can be understood as the scientific study of variation in the response of drugs due to heredity of individuals [2]. Though introduced quite early, pharmacogenomics caught attention in the year 1997, with advancement in the science of gene cloning and genome sequencing it was used in conjunction with pharmacogenetics [1]. However, the history of pharmacogenetics can be traced back to 510 B.C. when Pythagoras recognized the dangers of ingesting fava beans that resulted in fatal reaction in some individuals, and later on the reaction was attributed to the deficiency of G6PD in those individuals [3]. Establishment of the rules of heredity by Mendel in 1866 further shaped this field of research alongside publication of Garrod named "Inborn Errors of Metabolism". Other studies which further supported the science of pharmacogenetics include occurrence of unusual reactions to drugs on the basis of biochemical individuality studied by JBS Haldane, inborn variation in individuals for phenylthiocarbamide, atropine esterase activity in rabbits and occurrence of hemolytic disease in American soldiers of only African descent upon administration of the drug primaquine [3, 4]. Genetic deficiency of butyryl-cholinesterase (which resulted in death of individuals upon administration of succinylcholine injection for anesthesia) and N-acetyltransferase (responsible for metabolism of the drug isoniazid) further supported the concept of pharmacogenetics [4]. Further investigations also indicated presence of genetic differences at the level of human populations in addition to that of individuals. For example, Africans and Chinese have been found to be slow metabolizers for debrisoquine than Europeans and there is absence of alcohol metabolizing capacity in East Asians [4]. Knowledge of pharmacogenetics has thus given a new dimension to diagnosis, wherein physicians can individualize treatment for each patient, thereby producing better therapeutic response to therapy.

Genes play a vital role in the metabolism of many drugs; cytochromes P450 represent a major family of genes which are involved in regulation of metabolism of the drugs. Cytochromes P450 CYP3A4, CYP2C9, CYP2C19, and CYP2D6 are encoded by different genes and play a significant role in metabolism. A major fraction of the population lacks either of CYP2D6 or CYP2C19 because of the presence of inactivating genetic polymorphisms [1, 5]. Mere appearance of these inactive forms of variant alleles brings about the absence of activity affecting the metabolism of certain drugs metabolized by these enzymes. On the other side, a fraction of population have been found to have higher CYP2C19 or CYP2D6 activity than the normal, and are termed as ultrarapid metabolizers [6, 7]. Phase II metabolism involves conjugation reactions with sulphate, methyl, or glucuronic acid groups which are aided by certain enzymes and presence or absence of these enzymes affect Phase II metabolic reactions. For instance, it has been reported that polymorphism affects methylation of drug mercaptopurine (~0.3% of population lacks thiopurine methyltransferase) [8]. Certain genetic polymorphisms also cause structural alterations in drug targets apart from drug metabolism. Specific receptors on the surface of cells, enzymes, ion channels or transporters can be construed as drug targets. The gene VKORC1, encodes for Vitamin K epoxide reductase to which warfarin and other coumarin anticoagulants bind and has shown to exhibit extensive genetic polymorphism thus affecting drug response. This enzyme regulates regeneration of reduced vitamin K during the blood coagulation process [9]. Besides, indication of variation in drug metabolism and drug targets, pharmacogenetics also helps to discover adverse drug reactions due to exaggerated drug response, interaction with an inappropriate target or an inappropriate immune response to the drug [1].

2. Role of pharmacogenetics in diagnosis

Pharmacogenetics, including molecular genetics, has an essential role in the clinical management of diseases. Genetic testing has unfolded facts related to metabolism of drugs, and designing of personalized therapeutic regimens for safer and more efficient treatment with improved clinical outcomes. Practice of prescribing personalized medicine is gaining importance in healthcare as it helps to make therapeutic decisions based on individual characteristics, including genetic traits, quality of life, and environmental factors. Development in this field of science can provide important inputs which can be beneficial in diagnostics in cardiology (hemodynamics and electrophysiology), neurology, and oncology. Abundantly prescribed medications like Platelet aggregation inhibitors (PAIs), oral anticoagulants (OAs), antihypertensive and cholesterol-lowering drugs for cardiovascular disease, individual responses and efficacy can vary significantly due to genetic diversity. Genetics pharmacology and pharmacogenomics are genetically personalized guided therapies that optimize treatment and reduce toxicity. Genes have a significant influence on growth, development, health, and drug metabolism.

Human Genome Project (HGP) finished in 2003 helped to identify disease pathophysiology at the molecular level. With progress in bioinformatics and novel sequencing technologies for next-generation sequencing (NGS), sequencing of human genome has become easier, cost-effective and less time consuming. The National Human Genome Research Institute (NHGRI) has launched the DNA Elements Encyclopedia (ENCODE) to discover all functional sequences of the human genome [11]. Likewise, the Cancer Genome Atlas (TCGA) molecularly characterizes over 20,000 primary cancers, identifying and documenting the uniqueness of cancer types. 2.5 petabytes of genome, epigenome, transcriptome and proteomics data have been generated by TCGA to improve the ability to diagnose, treat and prevent cancer [10]. Sequencing disease-related mutant genes in many hereditary diseases and also, sequencing of target of disease-related genes can provide useful data in treatment of diseases. The PharmGKB base (https://www.pharmgkb.org/) and PGRN hub database (http://www.pgrn.org/) are coordinated with the Pharmacogenomics Research Network (PGRN) to impact treatment [11, 12]. The database from Pharmacogenomics PharmaGKB and Very Important Pharmacogene (VIP) link additional external resources to visualize genotypes, molecules, and clinical information of disease pathway representations to select the optimal regimen [11].

Adjustment of chemotherapeutic dosage according to genetic profile of individuals can also be achieved accordingly, which can help reduction of dose, side effects and toxicity. Genetic markers, HLA-B * 15:02 and HLA-B * 57:01 have been identified via HLA allelic testing of prescription drugs such as abacavir, and carbamazepine, respectively, but most genetic markers rarely reach such a dichotomy. The variability in clopidogrel response due to loss of CYP2C19 allele function is 12%. Heritable fluctuations are estimated to be 72%. This means that other genes are also involved in CYP2C19 variability in response to clopidogrel.

Additionally, the VKORC1 and CYP2C9 alleles account for less than 40% of dose variability upon administration of warfarin, further, rare mutations in genes have recently been reported, which may cause variation of unknown cause. Curtailed understanding of relationship of genetic effects and drug response can affect clinicians' and patients' confidence in genetic testing. It reduces clinical decision making for prediction of probabilities and possibilities. Pharmacological genomics-based clinical trials enhance drugs' development by establishing a correlation between genetic profile and patient outcome during the early stages of clinical trials. Phase III studies can be extended to individuals who have a genetic predisposition to safely and effectively use developmental drugs.

3. Pharmacogenetic tools to identify genetic variants

The three major approaches to detecting genetic mutations associated with drug responses are "candidate mutations", genome-wide association studies (GWAS), and whole-exome sequencing (WES). Genome-wide association studies (GWAS) is related to complete genome screening of hundreds of thousands of single nucleotide polymorphisms (SNPs) rather than candidate genes. Whole-exome sequencing identifies variants in the genome's protein-encoding regions and analyzes the genomic regions most likely to contain pathogenic variants and are being used frequently in pharmacogenetics of drug metabolism [13].

3.1 Genotyping in polymorphism

SNPs have become an essential marker for genetic research. Genotyping methods are mainly used to identify polymorphisms or SNPs that have great potential for developing new diagnostic markers that allow pharmaceutical and biotechnology research to identify genetic variation. Polymorphism can be detected via microfluidic devices and allows for very rapid fragment separation by high performance liquid chromatography and capillary electrophoresis, enabling detection of biomolecules of interest. Genotyping can be applied in the field of diagnostics, drug discovery, drug delivery, tissue engineering and bio-nanosensors ("lab-on-a-chip") [16]. High-speed, high-throughput SNP analysis using the innovative biochip nanotechnology based platform is an ideal technique for high-resolution mapping and population genome research and the development of electronic microarray platforms. Moreover, DMET Plus is a chip developed by Affymetrix that covers 1936 genetic variants (including SNPs and copy number variations) across 231 relevant genes. PharmaADME and "Core ADMEGene" comprises of a list of genes and genetic biomarkers that can be used to screen pharmacokinetic variability [14].

3.2 Candidate variants

Candidate gene studies help identify the frequency of genetic marker primarily SNPs present at a higher frequency among patients and healthy individuals. This hypothesis is based on identification of variants of particular genes of interest associated with a genotyped trait which will help in their quantitative assessment. Moreover, these candidate genes are selected for their functional role in pathogenesis or their linkage within chromosomal region. The candidate variants test determined through SNP test generally estimates the frequency of available disease-causing variants in individuals known as the non-functional mutations (indirect associations). These non-functional mutations exhibit strong linkage disequilibrium (LD) with direct association's functional mutations. Researchers have identified several variants of candidate genes such as VPS35, DNAJC13, HTRA2, NOS3, KCNS2, HAPLN4, USP46, SCN4A, TENM4, and FUS, probably under monogenic essential tremor conditions. However, their confirmation still requires a lot of independent research [15]. The genes NLRP2, FEZ2, CADM2, ANK3, NEK3, NEK7, TUBB, ANKRD1, and BRD2 are genetic mutations responsible for the development of the bipolar disorder (BD) and their detection in genetic tests will facilitate diagnosis. A better understanding of the genes and pathways involved is also needed to target genes that can improve treatment strategies. Further, GWAS and quantitative proteomics studies reveal the most significantly upregulated proteins in neural stem cells and mature neurons with brain damage [16].

3.3 Genome-wide association studies (GWAS)

Genome-wide association study (GWAS) is a technique that accurately and rapidly analyzes samples of the entire genome to determine genetic variation that causes the development of disease. It includes a human genome sequence for reference, a map of human genetic variation, and a computer database with advanced interpretation interfaces. Some of the genetic variations (DNA or genome) identified using GWAS have been shown in **Table 1**. This information will help in better diagnosis, prevention and treatment of common and complex diseases such as

Pharmacogenes	GWAS identified reference no	Structure/key points	Medical condition	Reference
Intronic HMGA2	rs1042725	Intracranial volume	Adult height Polymorphism HMGA2 influences the expression of the insulin-like growth factor 2 gene (IGF2) alongwith pleomorphic adenoma gene 1 (PLAG1)	[17]
Intronic CRHR1	rs17689882	Intracranial volume	Encodes corticotrophin-releasing hormone receptor.	[18]
Intonic GPCPD1	rs2618516	Occipital lobe surface area	Encode protein that hydrolyzes glycerophosphocholine	[19]
FBLN2	rs145212527	Hippocampal volume	Tissue organization and neuron differentiation	[20]
SNVs, LPL, LCAT, APOB, LDLRAP1, HCHOLA4, LDLR, APOB, PCSK	rs693, rs562338, rs506585, rs515135, rs1367117,rs757584	Genes facilitate receptor-mediated endocytosis, recycling, receptor regulation, biliary cholesterol excretion	Severe hypercholesterolemia	[21]
SLC12A3, CLCNKB, PN359k, PL94I, *CLCNKA, HNF1B*	NM_000339 NM_000085	Genes alter net renal sodium balance and blood pressure variation	Hypocalciuria and hypomagnesemia, Gitelman's syndrome (GS)	[22]
MYH7,TNNT2,TPMTNNI3, MYL2, MYBPC3, ACTC, MYL3	GTR000514111.4	Mutation in these genes may cause increased in TGF-β signaling in myocyte leading to fibrosis.	Familial Hypertrophic cardiomyopathy	[23]
FBN1	rs1036477 and rs2118181	Aortic aneurysm formation	Marfan's syndrome	[24]
NKX2–5, GATA-4, TBX5	rs2277923, rs28936670 rs368418329, rs56166237 rs6489957	The transcription factors for heart development and regulation	Atrial or ventricular septal defects, Congenital heart disease	[25]
NOTCH1	rs13300218-G rs3124592-A	NOTCH1 acts to suppress the default osteoblast mesenchymal flap	The bicuspid aortic valve, califi aortic valve disease	[26, 27]

Table 1.
GWAS identified pharmacogenes and its medical condition.

asthma, cancer, diabetes, heart disease and mental illness. Genome-wide association studies can also help in detection of the risk of drugs for type 2 diabetes, Parkinson's disease, heart disease, Crohn's disease, prostate cancer, and depression. Researchers conducted a genome-wide association study (GWAS) using participants from two groups: sick and similar people without illness. Their DNA samples are collected from participants by taking blood samples or cotton swabs by mouth. Certain genetic mutations occur more frequently in sick people as compared to non-sick people and thus, these variations are "related" to the disease. It has been observed that these genetic mutations identified in the human genome region are related to the cause of the disease. At the same time, the disease may not be directly linked to the cause of the disease, so, the mutation may be "marked" with the variant that actually causes the disease. Therefore, researchers often sequence DNA base pairs in that particular region of the genome to detect the actual genetic alterations that cause the disease to develop. The complete set of DNA, or each participant's genome, is purified and scanned on an automated laboratory machine by placing it on a small chip.

The National Center for Biotechnology Information (NCBI) has developed a genome-wide database of association studies. It collects data repositories related to various diseases known as databases of genotypes and phenotypes (dbGaP) accessible from the NCBI website (http://www.ncbi.nlm.nih.gov/entrez/query.fcgi?db=gap). The GWAS initiative was supported by the National Institutes of Health, Pfizer Global Research, and the Genome-wide Association Study (GAIN). GAIN is funding various GWAS studies on bipolar disorder, major depression, type 1 diabetic nephropathy, hyperactivity disorder, schizophrenia, and psoriasis at http://www.fnih.org.It can be found at work/past-programs/genetic-association-Information Network Gain. NIH Institute has also launched a genome-level related study at the National Institute of Cardiopulmonary Blood (NLBI) and a flamingham gene study in collaboration with Boston University School of Medicine for cardiovascular and other chronic disorders. Women's health studies have been contributed to the pharmacogenetics research network to investigate the effects of genes on osteoporosis, diabetes, and various responses of individuals to drugs, etc. The National Eye Institute and the National Institute of Neurological Disorders also pushed the Parkinson's disease stroke GWAS study.

3.4 Whole-exome sequencing (WES)

Whole exome sequencing, also known as next-generation sequencing (NGS), sequences the genome's protein regions. With this method, researchers can observe the effect of phenotypes by sequencing only the genome's coding regions. 2–3% of human exomes represent the entire genome, which is the root cause of approximately 85% of known disease-related mutants. Exome sequences can efficiently identify coding variants and find application in population genetics, genetic diseases, cancer research, and cost-effective alternatives to whole-genome sequencing. It also produces a more manageable dataset for faster and easier data analysis than the whole genome approach (a sequence of 4–5 Gb per exome versus about 90 Gb for the entire human genome). Exon sequencing detects exon encoding variants and extends targeted content to provide a more comprehensive view of gene regulation, including untranslated regions (UTRs) and microRNAs. The DNA library can be created in one day and requires only 4–5 Gb sequences per exome. Illumina DNA Prep with Exome Enrichment Kit, AmpliSeq for Illumina Exome Panel, TruSeq DNA Exome, TruSight One Sequencing Panels, Nextera DNA Exome, Library Prep Kit Selector are exome sequencing kits for analyzing coding regions of genomic variants.

In WES procedures, target regions with the fragmentation of genomic DNA are captured by hybridization using a solution of biotinylated oligonucleotide probe. The captured target sequence is isolated using streptavidin beads and subsequently amplified and sequenced after washing and elution. Their quantification helps in preparation of DNA libraries for high-quality whole-exome sequencing. Exome sequencing is useful in identifying Miller syndrome and rare Mendelian disease mutations. The NHLBI "Grand Opportunity" Exome Sequencing Project (GO-ESP) in association with Exome Aggregation Consortium (ExAC) helps to identify diseases associated with rare variants for the development of personalized medicine, and harmonizing patient-specific treatments.

4. Pharmacogenomic database

Pharmacogenetics is a field that provides information related to drug metabolizing enzymes, drug transporters, drug targets, and mutant genes that code for proteins necessary for drug response or toxicity. Next-generation sequencing is carried out by the rapid development of functional genomics that genetically analyzes the most essential mutations, gene copies, changes in the number of genomes and versatile arrays. These pharmacogenomics efforts help physicians prescribe safer and more effective treatments and personalized medications,. The joint clinical pharmacology genomics implementation consortium (CPIC, https: //cpicpgx.org/) project between the online resources PharmaGKB and Pharmacogenomics Research provides guidance on genetic testing to enhance and optimize drug therapy. In addition, the NIH-funded Implementing Genomics in Practice (IGNITE) initiative and the Dutch Pharmacogenomics Working Group (DPWG) in Europe have been developed with a focus on conducting and interpreting genetic testing to guide clinical decision-making. These consortia implement pharmacological genomics services in the clinic to update their knowledge according to pharmacological genomics guidelines. Some pharmacogenomic database and their attributes have shown in (**Table 2**).

4.1 The pharmacogenomics Knowledge Base (PharmGKB)

The Pharmacogenomics Knowledge Base (PharmGKB), funded by the National Institutes of Health and the Pharmacogenomics Research Network (PGRN), a joint research consortium, was developed at Stanford University to identify genetic mutations that affect drug responses [40]. The PharmGKB website (http://www.pharmgkb.org) contains genotypes, molecules and clinical knowledge integrated into the path representation, as well as additional external links to the all-important Pharmacogene (VIP). This is a web-based public repository of genotypic and phenotypic information related to the Pharmagenetics Knowledge Base (PharmGKB, http: //www.pharmgkb.org), which supports expression, storage, analysis, etc.) and distribution of pharmacogenetics data [37, 38]. PharmGKB aims to facilitate field research and facilitate the sharing of critical pharmacogenetic datasets. Pharmacological genomics can explain the various reactions (side effects and/or degree of positive response) to a drug due to the presence of specific alleles of the gene that explain the hereditary change. PharmGKB organizes data related to pharmacodynamics and response to medication, changes in pharmacokinetics, changes in molecular and cellular function assays, and changes in gene sequences. All datasets are categorized into these five sets and are also associated with related genes, drugs, and diseases.

Pharmacogenomic database	Attributes	Developed by	References
cBioPortal	Bioinformatics tools for visualization and gene-based analysis of cancer patients' molecular profiles and clinical attributes from large clinical trials.	Memorial Sloan Kettering Cancer Center (MSKCC) Computational Biology Center (cBio) is affiliated with The Cancer Genome Atlas (TCGA) and International Cancer Genomics Consortium (ICGC).	[28, 29]
CellMiner	Enables rapid retrieval of activity ratios of over 20,503 compounds, including 22,379 genes, 92 proteins, 360 microRNA transcripts, and 102 US Food and Drug Administration (FDA) approved drugs.	National Cancer Institute (NCI) Molecular Therapy Center (CMT) and Developmental Therapy Program (DTP)	[30, 31]
Connectivity Map	The CMAP 2.0 software identifies chemicals with similar gene profiling between the corresponding genes, or the gene signature previously identified as a general gene expression modification for one or more known compounds from the CMAP database. The software uses up-regulated and down-regulated query genes representing biological processes to detect both positive and negative connectivity compounds.	Broad Institute of MIT, Whitehead Institute and HarvardMedical School, Massachusetts	[32, 33]
MEDI and NDF-RT (Medication Reference Terminology and The National Drug File - Reference Terminology)	Database as a prescription drug resource to provide a range of unique diseases - drug combinations that suggest significant novelty potential	Developed by the US Department of Veterans Affairs Veterans Health Administration (VHA).	[34, 35]
SPHINX (Sequence Phenotype and Pharmacogenomics Integration Exchange)	This is an external database developed through the eMERGE project which, contrary to assisting doctors in prescribing, determines patient-specific information, mainly patient data and the new PGx from disease drug search engines.	The eMERGEseq initiative aims to identify rare variants. Partner Healthcare (two sequencing centres) with the Baylor Medical College Human Genomic Sequencing Center (HGSC) and Broad Institute has developed SPHINX to develop a series of high-impact genes, single nucleotide polymorphisms (SNVs), And the discovery of genomics by identifying and validating pathogenic variants.	[36]

Table 2.
Pharmacogenomic database.

4.2 The human cytochrome P450 (CYP) allele nomenclature website

The human cytochrome P450 allele nomenclature (CYP allele) (http://www.cypalleles.ki.se/) is a web-based analysis of CYP mutant genetic information with molecular and clinical effects. Most of the CYPs on the CYP allele website are polymorphic enzymes involved in the differentiation of foreign bodies but have endogenous functions. The website also contains information related NADPH cytochrome P450 oxidoreductase (POR), an electron donor of the CYP enzyme, which contains 29 CYP genes, so the POR allele is also a stellar allele nomenclature (POR*). This website covers the polymorphic alleles of NADPH cytochrome P450 oxidoreductase (POR) and 29 CYP enzymes' CYP2B6, CYP2C9, CYP2C19, and CYP2D6 genes. Each CYP allele contains information related to various alleles and their nucleotide changes, in vitro and in vivo molecular and functional effects [39].

4.3 The human arylamine N-acetyltransferase (NAT) gene nomenclature committee

Several genetic mutations related to human arylamine N-acetyltransferase (NATgene) in species, humans and other organisms have been identified and the allelic nomenclature for the gene has also been recognized. The committee will assist in the naming arylamine N-acetyltransferase and also its new arylamine N-acetyltransferase allele. The information will be accessible to the international scientific community via the Internet [40].

4.4 Transporter database (TP-search)

Homeostatic exchange between endogenous and extrinsic substances such as ions, small molecules, macromolecules and drugs and transport proteins (transporters) occurs at the systematic, organic, cellular and intracellular levels. Genomics, transcriptomics, and proteomics techniques for transporter genes in normal cellular processes and various pathologies have been integrated to develop the Human Transporter Database (HTD) (http://htd.cbi.pku.edu.cn) which indicate the relationship between expression patterns exhibited by transporter genes and polymorphisms and their ligands. Study on a human transporter involved in many fundamental biological processes, including oxidative phosphorylation and myocardial contraction, has shown the link between Mendel's laws and complex diseases. In particular, HTD serves as a well-organized interface to facilitate the research community to retrieve detailed molecular and genetic information for transporters and develop personalized medicine [41].

4.5 UGT alleles nomenclature page

The uridine diphosphate glucuronosyltransferase (UGT) enzyme involved in the glucuronidation of the target substrate makes foreign substances and other endogenous compounds water-soluble for renal excretion. The UGT Allele Nomenclature page describes the UGT1A1 haplotype. Developmental hyperbilirubinemia causes kernicterus or the accumulation of bilirubin in brain tissue. As a result of this, neurological damage occurs which is irreversible, resulting in severe disability or death. Bilirubin levels can be controlled by intensive phototherapy, the efficiency of which decreases with age, and the only alternative left is liver transplantation [42].

5. Role of nanotechnology in pharmacogenomics based diagnosis

Nanobio-labeling is an important tool in biomarker research that uses water-soluble, biocompatible, fluorescent and stable nanomaterials to label cells. Molecular biomarkers can be used in designing of personalized medicine for diagnosis and treatment, identifying cellular changes at the DNA, RNA, biotransformer or protein level. Nanotechnology based devices can potentially screen disease biomarkers at high speed. The tools are developed by identifying biomarkers very specific for the disease that can lead to diagnostic tests. These nanobiotechnology-based diagnostic methods, which use direct DNA and protein analysis, can improve speed, accuracy and sensitivity over traditional molecular diagnostic techniques. Nanobiotechnology supports molecular diagnostics, and integration of diagnostics and therapeutics (theranostics) which accelerates personalized medicine [43]. Theranostic applications can help provide optimal treatments and characterize human genomic mutations between populations [44].

According to a report published by Grand View Research, Inc., the global market for pharmacogenomics (theranostics and complementary diagnostics) is expected to reach $18.3 billion by 2025. These approaches help provide cost-effective treatment and add value to the process, of development. The benefits of using these tests for disease risk prediction, patient stratification, and treatment response monitoring, over traditional methods are expected to provide significant progress in this market [45].

The role of genetics plays a vital role in theranostics, which provides successful and cost-effective therapeutic.

Pharmacological genetics, proteomics, and biomarker profiling based diagnosis using nanotechnology based platforms like liposomes, dendrimers, macromolecular nanoparticles, metal nanoparticles, quantum dots, and carbon nanotubes is providing vital information regarding disease pathology and its treatment. Quantum dots are stable particles which can be used as molecular labels to study the size and span of metastasis besides, predicting early signs of cancer and tracking the effectiveness of drugs targeting the disease. Genzyme Corporation has discovered EGFR mutation detection kits that can be used to diagnose non-small cell lung cancer (NSCLC) [46].

6. Multiple genes interactions on treatment response

Multiple genetic interactions also termed as polygenic inheritance interconnects biological processes and their functional relationships that cause phenotypic deviations and multiple genetic mutations [47]. A retrospective study of 108 Chinese patients with metastatic gastric cancer found nine genes involved in DNA repair (ERCC1, ERCC2, and XRCC1), detoxification of oxaliplatin (GSTP1 and GSTT1), and fluoropyrimidine metabolism (MTHFR) and these can be used to predict clinical response and survival [48]. Similarly, the Mayo Clinic has issued drug-gene pair alerts on 17 drug-gene pairs: Abacavir HLA-B*57:01, Allopurinol HLA-B*58:01, Carbamazepine HLA-B*15:02 and HLA-A*31:01, Citalopram CYP2C19,Clopidogrel CYP2C19, Codeine CYP2D6, Escitalopram CYP2C19, Fluoxetine CYP2D6, Fluvoxamine CYP2D6, Paroxetine CYP2D6, Simvastatin SLCO1B1, Tacrolimus CYP3A5,Tamoxifen CYP2D6, Thiopurines TPMT, Tramadol CYP2D6, Venlafaxine CYP2D6,Warfarin CYP2C9 and VKORC1 which will help physicians treat patients on the basis of the genetic test in response to the alert. These evidence-based guidelines were established by the Consortium for the implementation of clinical pharmacogenomics [49].

7. Pharmacogenomic based diagnosis of cancer

Various cancer portals have been developed for tumor gene profiling and are serving as a powerful tool for discovering and implementing personalized cancer treatments. Large-scale translational bioinformatics and cancer genomics platforms use multi-omics datasets to provide insight into genomic alternations and precision medicine strategies. Development in tools for statistical, mathematical and computational modeling help collect genomic information for molecular profiling, clinical responses to drugs, research on clinical trials, and identification and development of innovative therapies. Transcriptome data from melanoma exsons pretreated with ipilimumab was studied to study the effect of pretreatment on activity of tumor-specific new antigens including mutation loading, new antigen loading, and cytolysis in the tumor microenvironment [50]. The Cancer Genome Atlas (TCGA) study performs molecular subtyping of the breast, colorectal and endometrial cancers. Furthermore, TP53 inactivation, MYC proliferation and dysregulated cell cycle checkpoints have been demonstrated through TCGA studies [51]. The role of pharmacogenomics is more pronounced in oncology as compared to other diseases and is indicating that inherited differences in genes affect the body's response to medications. Pharmacogenetics has revolutionized cancer treatment by genotyping patients in clinical settings that promote the best chemotherapeutic regimens and drug doses with maximum efficacy and minimal risk of toxicity. The Pharmacology Genomics Resources (PREDICT) program for enhanced decisions in care and treatment initiated by Vanderbilt University has simplified consistent dosing. Pharmacogenomic data identified for application in diagnosis and treatment has been shown in (**Table 3**).

S.no	Pharmacogenomic data	Diagnostic/Treatment Protocol	Reference
1.	Dihydropyrimidine dehydrogenase (DPYD) genotype and fluoropyrimidine dosing	The DPYD gene sequencing and it's variant has been significantly analyzed by polymorphism (G to A intron 14 (inv14 + 1G > A or DPYD*2A; exon skipping mutation). Dosing of fluoropyrimidine depends on genotyping of DPYD, a rate-limiting enzyme for fluoropyrimidine catabolism.	[52]
2.	Methylenetetrahydrofolate reductase (MTHFR)	Methylenetetrahydrofolate reductase (MTHFR) is an essential regulator of folic acid and homocysteine metabolism. In epilepsy, the concentration of 5-methyl-THF in CSF should be monitored. The CSF concentration of 5-methyl-THF is significantly reduced in most early-onset patients due to restricted transport of folic acid through the blood-CSF barrier and increased demand for choline for meningeal biosynthesis resulting in severity of the neurologic symptoms in MTHFR deficiency.	[53]
3.	Thiopurine S-methyltransferase (TPMT) and thiopurine dosing	The prodrugs azathioprine, 6-mercaptopurine (6-MP) and thioguanine (TG) are inactivated by TPMT and methylated to produce TG active nucleotide (TGN). 6-MP is biotransformed to methylthionosin 5-prime monophosphate, which causes inhibition of de novo purine synthesis and can cause toxic effects. TPMT gene genotyping is used for thiopurine dose assessment in myelosuppression. TPMT test is mandatory before use of mercaptopurine in childhood leukemia.	[54]

S.no	Pharmacogenomic data	Diagnostic/Treatment Protocol	Reference
4.	Uridine diphosphate glucuronosyl transferase (UGT) genotype and irinotecan	Irinotecan is activated to SN-38. UGT1A1 family is involved in glucuronidation of SN-38 and bilirubin. Variation in the number of TA dinucleotide repeats in the TATA element of the UGT1A1 promoter region, is associated with reduced gene expression as well as diminished enzyme activity	[55]
5.	Glutathione S-transferases gene polymorphism and platinum compounds	Glutathione S-transferase (GST) constitutes a family of enzymes involved in detoxification of foreign bodies', including cisplatin-based chemotherapy. Genetic polymorphisms in GST have shown altered efficacy or toxicity in patients with NSCLC (more specifically GSTP1 is associated with improved response to therapy)	[56]
6.	ATP-binding cassettes (ABCB1, ABCC2, ABCG2)	The ABCB1 gene encodes P-glycoprotein. Overexpression of this glycoprotein leads to resistance to specific anti-cancer therapies. There are two synonymous SNPs (C1236T for exon 12 and C3435T for exon 26) and one non-synonymous SNP (G2677T for exon 2), which appear to be regulated by MDR1 * 2 haplotypes, P-glycoprotein upregulation and drugs. ABCG2 (Breast Cancer Resistant Protein) and ABCC2 are involved in irinotecan's metabolism and alter the properties of irinotecans.	[57]
7.	X-ray cross complementing group 1 (XRCC1)	XRCC1 is a DNA repair protein. It is encoded by the XRCC1 gene in humans. SNPs (1301 G > A; Arg399Gln) result in mutations in base excision ability and increased cancer risk. Negative expression of XRCC1 makes tumors more sensitive to platinum-based chemotherapy. Detection of XRCC1 expression in patients with gastric cancer can provide clinical guidance in choosing the optimal adjuvant for therapy.	[58]

Table 3.
Pharmacogenomic data identified for application in diagnosis and treatment.

8. Pharmacogenomic diagnosis for cardiac diseases

Clopidogrel is used in the acute coronary syndrome patients, exhibits variable response in patients due to *2 loss-of-function variant in CYP2C19 as it encodes hepatic cytochrome P-450 2C19 enzyme which is important for clopidogrel bioactivation. Similarly, interindividual variation in response to warfarin is due to polymorphisms in VKORC1 and CYP2C9 and has been led to revision of dosing guidelines for patients by USFDA. Variant of SLCO1B1, which encodes a hepatic uptake transporter, is associated with risk of myopathy with high-dose (80 mg/d) simvastatin [59]. Genetic mutations in thiopurine S-methyltransferase (TPMT), an enzyme that metabolizes azathioprine, result in higher concentration of the azathioprine active metabolite. Combining the immunosuppressant azathioprine and the enzyme thiopurine S-methyltransferase, is used to prevent heart transplant rejection [60]. Sufficiently robust and predictive genetic information can be used to guide clinical decisions [61]. The European Pharmacogenetics of Anticoagulant Therapy (EU-PACT) found a significant association between PGx-guided warfarin dosing [62]. The genes most strongly associated with beta-blocker response are the β-1 adrenergic receptor (ADRB1), the α-2C adrenergic receptor (ADRA2C) and the G protein-coupled receptor kinase-5 gene (GRK5). The ADRB1 gene has two common non-synonymous single nucleotide polymorphisms, p.Ser49Gly and p.Arg389Gly, associated with different responses to beta-blockers in hypertension and coronary heart disease [59]. The genome aggregation database maintains archives the various gene variants. Guidelines for 27 drug-gene pair has been issued by Pharmagenetics Implementation Consortium, and includes data related to drug metabolizer phenotypes. (extensive metabolizer/slow metabolizer), poor/ultrafast metabolizer, expected rapid metabolizer with a particular diplotype, expected effect size, availability of alternative therapies, and results of drug ineffectiveness or toxicity [63].

9. Pharmacogenomic diagnosis for brain disorders

Only 30–40% patients with central nervous system disorders respond conventional drugs. Around 60–90% of variability in drug response is due to pharmacogenetic and pharmacogenomic factors. Approximately 60–80% of CNS drugs are metabolized via enzymes of the CYP gene superfamily. Neuroleptics are the major substrates of CYP1A2, CYP2D6 and CYP3A4 enzymes. Antidepressants are essential substrates for CYP1A2, CYP2B6, CYP2C19, CYP2D6, CYP3A4 and benzodiazepines are vital substrates of CYP2C19, CYP2D6 enzymes. Adoption of genomic medicine have proven to be prognostic tools to accelerate diagnostic accuracy in CNS disorders' etiology and develop novel biomarkers to personalize treatments via pharmacogenetic and pharmacogenomic procedures for drug development and clinical practice [64].

10. Role of nanotechnology and pharmacogenomics in the treatment of diseases

Advances in molecular pharmacology, genomics and nanotechnology are providing enriching clinical results by meticulously highlighting pathogenesis pathways, empowering the capacity for clinical diagnosis, and improving the outcome of drug delivery [65]. Supported by the sophisticated target-guided nanodevices, the intricate genomic information is being incorporated into clinical practice to evaluate complex diseases such as cardiovascular diseases, type 2 diabetes, asthma, cancer and degenerative disorders [66]. Presence of unique genetic variants has been found to be instrumental in predisposing particular individuals to the onset and development of diseases. Nanotechnology based drug delivery systems have developed specialized technical frameworks for the exploitation of genomic knowledge, so as to reduce the risk of disease initiation and progression and drug toxicity [67]. Pharmacogenomics highlights the interplay of the role of genes in disease etiology, disease pathophysiology, disease biomarkers, drug targets, drug effects, and the fate of drugs inside the body. The integrated application of pharmacogenomics and nanotechnology will provides better therapeutic outcomes with minimized side effects and adverse drug reactions during therapy [68].

10.1 Pharmacogenomics

Pharmacogenomics emerged as a science which highlighted the differences in drug response to differences in genetic makeup in particular populations/various ethnic groups. It is the science of genetic polymorphism (genetic variance) that is responsible for variability in drug response and is used as a useful method to assess the association of disease-gene, and gene-drug on drug response based on the human genome. Drugs are formulated and designed to counteract medical conditions and cure ailments, but drugs often fail to demonstrate their beneficial impact in certain patients, resulting in adverse drug events. This drug response variability may be due to genetic differences [69]. The research of hereditary variability in drug receptors or target pathways, heterogeneity in genes that encode drug-metabolizing enzymes or drug transporters, and genetic variation in genes that indirectly affect drug reaction are part of Pharmacogenomics. The main objective of pharmacogenomics is to recognize how genetic differences affect therapeutic efficacy and this knowledge can be used experimentally to personalize the selection of medications and their doses to improve efficacy and safety.

Pharmacogenetic tests have historically focused on specific candidates selected based on our understanding of the pharmacokinetics of the drug, and drug response variability found in patients receiving the medication. Initially, family experiments were used to determine the hereditary existence of inter-individual variations in the disposition of drug or effect of medications, which was then used to understand the genetic cause for monogenic traits. Pharmacogenomics can be seen as a wider approach to elucidate the abundance of genes that are important to pharmacology, including the implications of genetic differences in single genes, the relationship between genes in diverse pharmacological pathways, the phenotype that arises from these differences, and the impact of the phenotype on drug response. Its main characteristics are high-throughput genomic studies in conjunction with their significance to particular drug responses only as target phenotype (i.e., sequence variants in DNA, gene exposition analysis, etc.). The structural and functional genomics analysis (**Figure 1**) can be used to understand the use of therapeutic drugs for increased efficacy (with reduction in toxicity) for dosage personalization and new drug development [70]. The structural pharmacogenomics explores the structural difference between individuals' genes while functional genomics evaluate the functional modifications induced by structural variation in the genome. Variations in genes are responsible for the variation in particular functional process inside the body via change in the nature of protein synthesized. Any disorder or deformity may also result due to these functional changes. Both structural and functional pharmacogenomics are effective in predicting, recognizing genetic markers of disease, and planning and optimizing drug therapy in the treatment of that disease [71].

Extremely penetrating monogenic features are several of the genetic polymorphisms characterized to date that affect drug reaction in humans: hereditary variations in a specific gene have such a significant effect on the pharmacokinetics or pharmacodynamics of a drug that cross changes in one gene have a clinically relevant effect on drug response. "These are pharmacogenetics' "low-hanging fruit". However, certain proteins decide the efficacy of certain medications, and hybrid genetic polymorphisms can be identified to determine therapeutic efficacy of several genes along with nongenetic factors. Therefore, new methods are required to classify the appropriate genes, genetic polymorphisms, mechanisms, and processes and; their association with a given drug. The different techniques currently being utilized are genome-wide haplotype analysis, gene regulation tests and proteomic techniques, as well as "candidate gene" approaches focused on

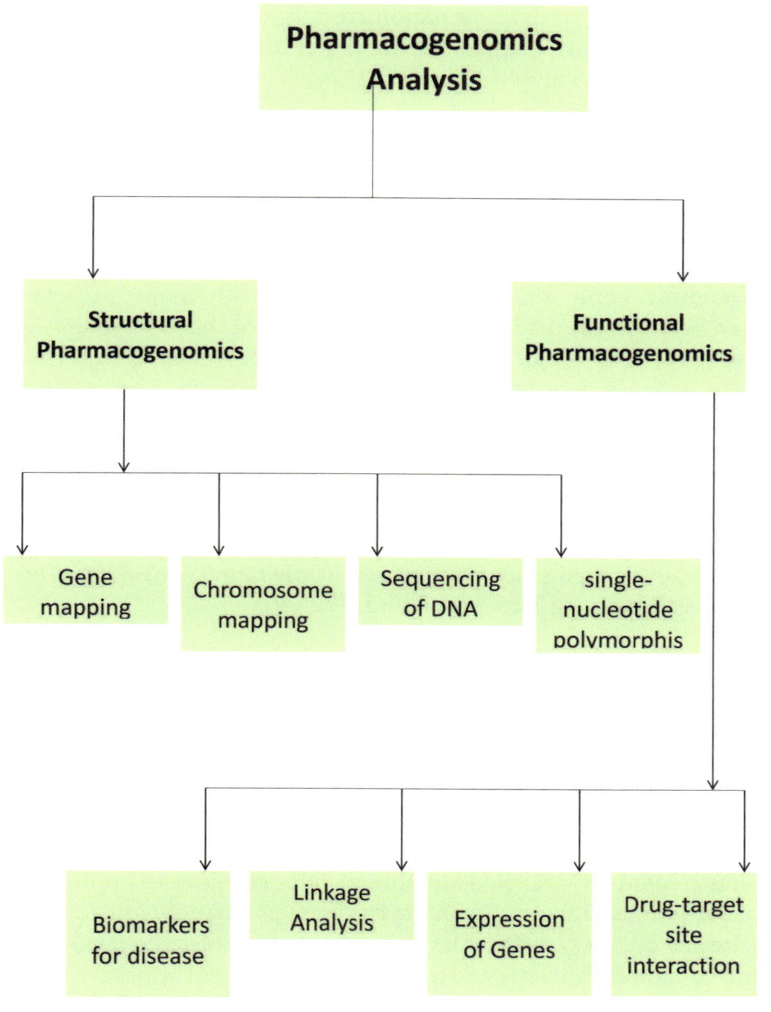

Figure 1.
Structural and functional pharmacogenomics analysis.

established pharmacokinetic and pharmacodynamic considerations. These methods are likely to be important for studies that seek to elucidate polygenic determinants of drug response, with emerging predictive and biological (pathway) models and quantitative genotyping in certain target tissues. Broad clinical trials with uniformly treated and routinely characterized patients, high-throughput genomic approaches, and advanced bioinformatics simulations would entail the clinical validity of these polygenic models. These experiments aim to create a new range of molecular diagnostics (i.e. genotypes) that can be used to enhance drug delivery by reducing toxicity and maximizing efficacy [72].

Nanotheranostics is the field where pharmacogenomics is used in the delivery of drugs for personalized medicines. It is a hybrid of drug therapies and diagnostics. Pharmacogenomics provides an excellent method to quantify several parameters relating to the disorder and its severity, together with treatment, so that medicine can be tailored on the basis of an individual's genotype. Nanotechnology offers a possibility for the development and design of therapeutic strategies, which are capable of concurrently detecting genetic biomarkers for disease along with ongoing drug therapy. Nanotechnological materials such as gold-based nanomaterials, magnetic nanomaterials, polymeric nanomaterials, carbon-based nanomaterials, silica-based nanomaterials, composite nanomaterials and quantum dots may be used to build such drug delivery systems [73, 74].

10.2 Role of Pharmacogenomics in the identification of drug targets

Structural Pharmacogenomics aims to recognize and verify disease-relevant targets for therapeutic activity (target biomarker) like the EGFR signaling system, PI3K, RAF, MAPK, KRAS AKT markers for various forms of cancers. Pharmacogenomics compares the target biomarkers with disease processes to create a connection between the disease and the biomarker of the experiment, which then helps to define the drug molecule for such a target [75, 76]. Specific genome targets like enzymes, drug carriers, proteins, nucleic acids, chromosomes, cell surface proteins, ion channels, and other bio-molecules contributing to the pathophysiology of the disease have been provided by human genome sequencing. Such possible causes to the pathophysiology of the disease can serve as target sites for drug action (druggable targets). Thus, the pharmacogenomics concept can be used in target recognition, genotyping, structural elucidation, and target confirmation that improve safety and efficacy of medicines. Sequencing of the target genes can be used in the discovery and validation of lead compounds [77, 78].

10.3 Nanotechnology towards making possibility of personalized medicine

Nanotechnology is the development and utilization of materials, devices and processes by manipulating matter at the nanometer range, i.e. at the level of atoms, molecules, and supermolecular structures. The application of nanotechnology in life sciences is in molecular diagnostics, drug discovery, drug delivery and nanomedicine development. The combination of nanotechnology with personalized medicine has created unparalleled and unique opportunities to improve the treatment of many serious diseases. Medicine has been profoundly impacted by this concept over the last decades, shifting its attention to the molecular level under which, applications of nanotechnology as a quickly emerging field appear to fit needs on this size scale. In this reference, nanoparticles offer unique benefits in the design of nanomedicine due to their small size, flexibility, increased surface-to-volume ratio and multi-purpose ligand surface modification in order to obtain targeting of cells/tissues. Nanomedicine is also meant to offer immediate, precise and efficient diagnosis and treatment. In this way, the balance between maximum therapeutic efficacy and lower toxicity is significantly promoted [79, 80].

As the nanomedicine market has expanded exponentially, the most promising technologies and applications for personalized medicine can be identified. Individuality of a person is often expressed in his pathophysiology. In the same extent genes define, the identity of an individual, genetic heterogeneity that can identify the disease phenotype and its drug response. It is reported that each drug has different effects on different types of peoples. Whether in terms of efficacy and safety of these drugs, they show differential behavior due to the complex nature and heterogeneity of individuals (both patients and diseases). With a sound and detailed knowledge of genomics and proteomics and the development of a novel and innovative technology and patient-based molecular profiling, the promise of nanomedicine has opened the path to the future of personalized medicine [80, 81].

Personalized medicine literally means prescribing of particular medications that are ideally suited to the person. Personalized medicine is the perfect way to incorporate modern biotechnology into medicine in order to improve understanding of disease pathomechanism, molecular identification and clinical application.

Nowadays, nanotechnology and genomics fuel expertise and creative practices, allowing both pharmacological strategies and therapeutics measures to be implemented on a personal basis, i.e. designing personalized medications (Innovative Drugs), improving targeted drug delivery and pharmacotyping techniques to the clinical environment for diagnosis and treatment of disease as shown in (**Figure 2**). "Pharmacotyping" is characterized as the prescription drug mechanism by which clinical and genotyping data are used to instruct physicians to design drug dose regimens for particular patients. These approaches require a comprehensive genetic and molecular history of each patient, which leads to the discovery of specific biomarkers that might influence the progression of the disease and the response to treatment. Personalized medicine is also not only restricted to the study of biomarkers and genetic polymorphisms, but also depends on the development of disease identification techniques and estimation of therapeutic responses [73]. Thus, understanding

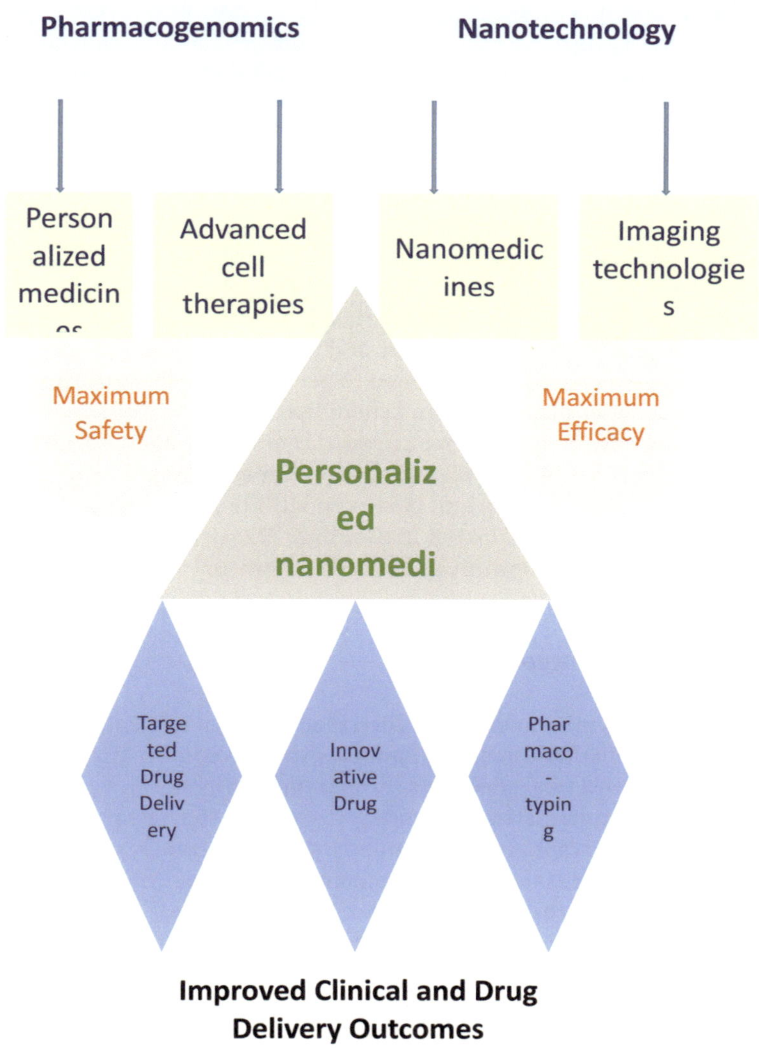

Figure 2.
Integrated approach of nanotechnology and pharmacogenomics to improve safety and efficacy of drugs.

of nanotechnology and genomics could handle the disease and drug response of patients in the form of personalized medicines. In addition, recent developments in nanotechnology have certainly provided the perfect environment for the emergence of personalized medicine as the new approach in the diagnosis of diseases and drug therapy.

10.4 Nanoparticles in personalized medicine

Because of their exploratory features, nanoparticles facilitate the molecular targeting of medicines. Recent studies offered detailed information on the relationship of NPs with biological processes in order to promote their use for nanotheranostics diagnosis, imaging and drug delivery. Today, nanotheranostics have been developed to monitor transcription and translation of genes, recognize cancer cells, control the proliferation of T cells, and manage blood sugar levels. Moreover, blood urea levels can be detected by an implant and normal levels can be restored. Another implant was created for artificial insemination that injects bull spermatocytes into the bovine ovary by identifying luteinizing hormone levels, especially during ovulation. Any disorder can be treated at the cellular and molecular level by detecting particular biochemical parameters [79]. While several experiments have been performed, relatively few pharmaceutical drug products have been developed as nanotherapeutics in the pharmaceutical market, indicating the uncertainty of formulating active compounds in these formulations. A PEGylated liposome doxorubicin medication called Doxil, approved for therapeutic use by the FDA, is the most popular example of nanoparticle technology for clinical use. The principle of PEGylation was first developed as a means for recombinant protein drugs to improve their circulation and stability. Another FDA approved effective nanoparticle application is Abraxane, in which paclitaxel is formulated with albumin. In an attempt to merge nanoscale therapeutic and diagnostic modalities, separate nanotheranostic agents have been designed to provide flexible platforms for the simultaneous delivery of diagnostics and therapeutics [73].

However, many new materials have arisen as theranostic agents such as gold nanoparticles, carbon nanotubes, metal organic frameworks and iron oxide nanoparticles; problems of safety and bio - compatibility and unspecified tolerance and toxicity need to be evaluated in the clinic. Regardless of these drawbacks, nanotheranostics seem very optimistic to develop personalized medicine [79].

11. Personalized nanomedicines

Personalized nanomedicine may be described as the management of a patient's disease or drug response by the use of nanomedicine in combination with clinical and molecular expertise (e.g. genomics, proteomics, epigenomics and metabolomics) as well as bioinformatics techniques to produce the best possible medical treatment for that person. In addition, by integrating nanotechnology and genomics expertise, personalized nanomedicine may create enhanced profiles for particular demographics and particular patients for prognosis, diagnosis and drug therapy, as well as surveillance through medical science and clinical management (**Table 4**) [81].

The combination of nanotheranostics with pharmacogenomics will take us to the next level of therapeutics. On one hand, the concept of pharmacogenomics is the latest model research, which has tremendous implications throughout the field of medical science and drug development at genomic and molecular level; moreover, a great deal of work is needed to investigate the maximum capabilities of

Advantages of Personalized Nanomedicines
Personalized nanomedicine is in nano-scale size range
Personalized nanomedicine offers tunability and flexibility
Offers possibility of using labile substances such as siRNA
The active concepts of personalized nanomedicine: encapsulation and safety
Targeted delivery to organs/ tissues/ cell compartments
Probability of responding to a need of specific patient group
Adapting patterns of treatment to each patient (e.g., dosage, frequency, etc.)

Table 4.
Advantages of personalized nanomedicines.

this method in the clinical field. Theranostics, on the other hand, is the technique of early phase diagnosis or disease pathogenesis, combined with concurrent treatment based on a single unit operation diagnosis profile. This not only increases patient health with optimum clinical performance, but also saves significant amounts of money by minimizing excessive care costs. This approach is of significantly more useful in the treatment of life-threatening chronic diseases like cancer, hypertension, Alzheimer disease, and can be implemented to many other ailments [68].

11.1 Personalized nanomedicine in the treatment of cancer

The advancement of personalized nanomedicine is a useful technique in the cancer therapy. Personalized oncology is raising new prospects for the elimination of cancer incidence by specifically targeting anticancer medicines to cancerous cells, target areas on the cell surface and inside the tumor microenvironment. Nanooncology has succeeded in improving the specificity and efficiency of cancer therapies, both by promoting the development and distribution of medications and by reducing clinical toxicity and serious incidents [82]. Personalization of cancer treatment is focused on a deeper knowledge of the pathogenesis at the molecular scale and nanomedicine can play a significant role in this direction. Several nanobiotechnology-relevant components of personalized cancer treatment are given in (**Figure 3**) [83]. Nanobiotechnology has the ability to enhance early cancer diagnosis and enhance personalized cancer treatment. Molecular diagnostics is the most important aspect of personalized medicine, and nanobiotechnology can play a significant role in its refinement [84].

Dendrimers are a class of nanoscale, core-shell, three-dimensional structures that can be synthesized precisely for a variety of uses. Specialized methods in chemistry allow detailed control over the dendrimer's physical and chemical properties. They are most effective in the delivery of drugs, but they can also be used to produce new pharmaceuticals with emerging technologies. With several therapeutic target, polyvalent dendrimers interact simultaneously. They can be transformed into new-targeted therapeutics for cancer. Using complementary DNA oligonucleotide primers, dendrimers may be covalently linked to various bio-functional groups, such as folic acid, to create clustered molecules attacking cancer cells that overexpress the high affinity folate receptor [85]. Endothelial $\alpha v\beta 3$-Integrin-targeted paramagnetic nanoparticles are being used to identify very limited angiogenesis area linked with tumors of nascent melanoma [86]. Nanobodies (Ablynx) are the smallest intact antigen binding fragments that have the full antigen binding capacity of natural heavy-chain antibodies. Nanobodies are prospective era of antibody-based treatments as well as diagnostic tools for diseases like cancer.

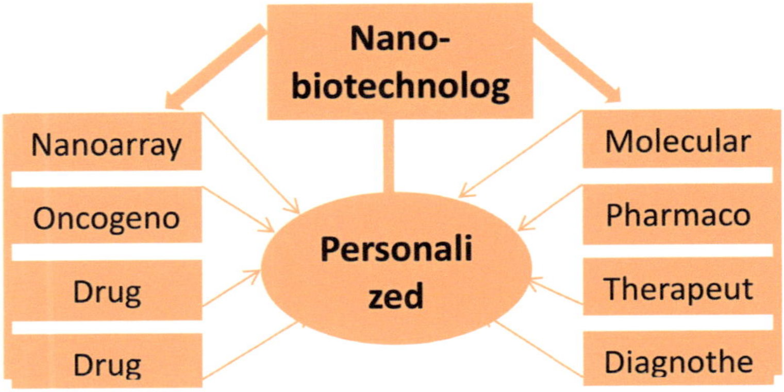

Figure 3.
Function of nanobiotechnology for personalized cancer treatment.

Nanobodies have a relatively high specificity and low endogenous toxicity. They can tackle therapeutic targets that are not readily detected by traditional antibodies such as enzyme active sites. Nanobodies have the ability to be produced as personalized cancer therapies [87]. Nanotechnology is revolutionizing the treatment of cancer as it can alter its diagnosis, clinical path, and prognosis. Before treatment, cancer molecular profiling may be extremely prognostic and predictive of clinical responses or recurrence, encouraging the most effective treatment to be prescribed with each specific cancer.

11.2 Personalized nanomedicine for targeting CNS diseases

Central nervous system (CNS) disorders are increasingly worldwide due to changing demographics. Three factors make this field especially challenging as, pathogens are slowly evolving and impossible to diagnose early or anticipate, response to medication is highly dependent on the individual patient and always needs to be personalized, and drugs must pass the blood brain barrier [88]. Therapeutic agents commonly used to treat CNS diseases have shown considerable efficacy. However, the failure of these medicines to pass the blood–brain barrier (BBB) and the inefficacy of technology to ensure localized delivery of drugs in disease-specific areas of the brain have impeded full CNS disease management. Nanoparticle- based targeted drug delivery to the brain will play a significant component in designing personalized treatment of neurological disorders by enhancing molecular diagnosis and pathomechanisms. For CNS drug delivery system, different types of nanoparticles (gold, silica, hydrogels, liposomes, magnetic nanoparticles, etc.) have been investigated. Such examples of the use of personalized treatment-based nanotechnology to treat CNS diseases are as follows: [89].

Gene silencing technologies focusing on small interfering RNA (siRNA) have shown great potential for the treatment of brain-associated diseases. However, successful and systemic delivery of siRNA to the brain appears difficult due to biological challenges such as enzymatic depletion, short-lived circulation, blood–brain barrier (BBB), relatively low tissue penetration, cell endocytosis, and cytosolic transport. Nanotechnology provides an interesting opportunity to overcome these problems in the delivery of siRNA to brain in combination with chemical and biological alteration strategies [90].

Alzheimer's disease (AD) is a major public health concern worldwide. The challenge in treating the disease is partly attributed to the uncertainty of the signs and symptoms, the still limited understanding of its pathways and the presence of latent, asymptomatic, condition. While several drugs are constantly screened in clinical trials for the treatment of Alzheimer's disease, the unpredictable patient response and often-serious adverse effects provide space for development for personalized nanomedicine [91]. In a study involving AD, the brain region was irradiated with low gigahertz electromagnetic fields after binding of gold nanoparticles to β-amyloid plaques. The energy level was quite low for healthy cells to be affected. This study can be used effectively in the treatment of CNS disorder involving protein aggregation [92].

A "nanozyme" consists of a composition of the nanoparticle, an enzyme and a moiety for recognition. In Parkinson's disease (PD), oxidative stress degrades the main dopaminergic receptors in the brain resulting in inflammation. It is also assumed that catalyzing the enzyme might be beneficial in therapy. Nanozyme, encapsulating catalase, and macrophages extracted from bone marrow linked to a recognition moiety, when administered, showed that navigation of the nanozyme into the region of brain's inflammation. As a result, better distribution and improved bioavailability are achieved through the BBB [93].

11.3 Personalized nanomedicine for cardiovascular diseases

The development of cardiovascular diagnosis is now being influenced by nanosystems that can both detect and treat disease with a targeted delivery system. Nanotechnology has the ability to significantly accelerate the acceptance of personalized medicines in area of cardiovascular research by allowing production of fast, multimode point-of-care identification of single nucleotide polymorphisms (SNPs). This will, in essence, include information on the dangers associated with the progression of particular coronary disorders and pharmacogenetic advice on appropriate treatment for individual patients. In order to be clinically effective, the ideal method would need to be convenient, reliable, capable of simultaneous calculation of multiple genotypes and capable of conducting the full study without user intervention [94]. The different approaches to nanomedicine used in the form of nanocardiology have been mentioned in (**Figure 4**).

The possibility of cardiovascular procedures for the treatment of cardiovascular disorders appears to be interconnected with nanosystems capable of providing pathological diagnosis and treatment by means of changeable and regulated targeted systems. The dual potential of nanoparticles for visualization and selective distribution of therapeutic drugs to patients with cardiovascular disease would be a great opportunity for personalized medicine. By combining target drug delivery and molecular imaging with magnetic resonance imaging, the functions of serials by expressing epitope can be identified. At the desired target, monitoring and treatment validation will clear the way for individual treatments [95].

11.4 Personalized nanomedicine for bone disorders

Osteoporosis is the most common metabolic bone disorder, and osteoporosis susceptibility genes (ESR1, LRP5, SOST, OPG, RANK and RANKL) are involved in three biological pathways: the estrogen endocrine pathway, the Wnt/β-catenin signaling pathway and the RANK/RANKL/osteoprotegerin (OPG) pathway [96]. Estrogen plays an essential role in bone biology through binding to two different estrogen receptors (ESRs), ESR1 and ESR2. Women's Health Initiative performed a randomized controlled trial of hormone therapy, in which oral conjugated 0.625 mg equine estrogen with or without 2.5 mg medroxyprogesterone acetate was administerd and showed significant reduction in postmenopausal risk of osteoporosis [97]. Vascular endothelial growth factor A (VEGFA), is highly expressed

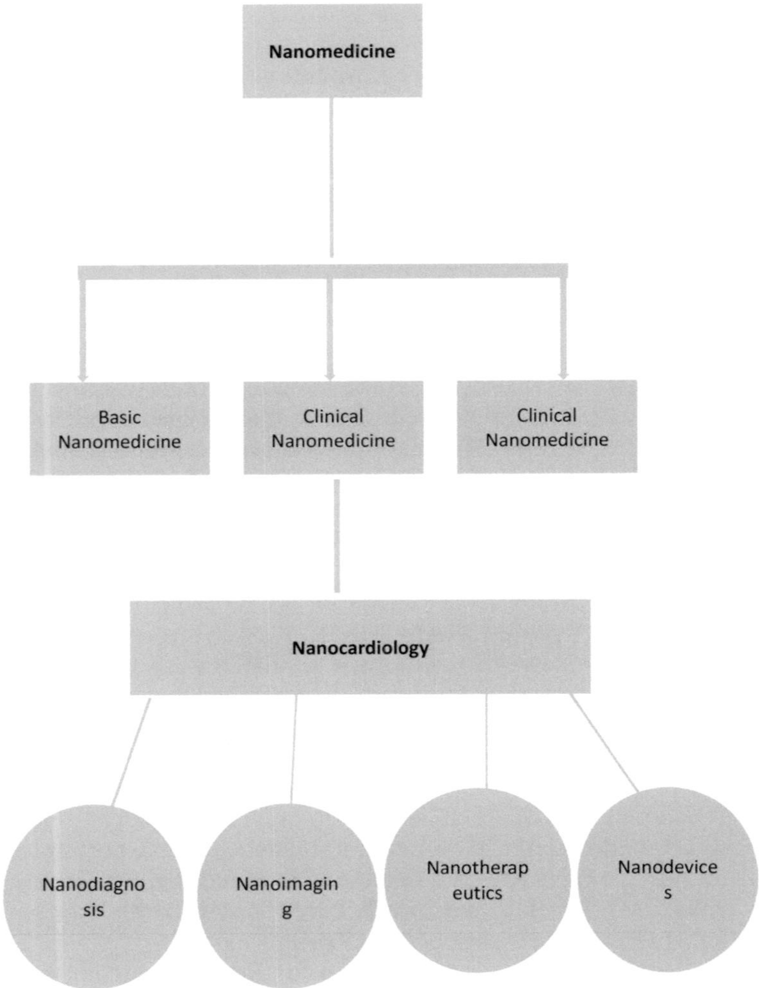

Figure 4.
Nanomedicine in the context of nanocardiology for cardiovascular disease management.

in osteocarcinoma (OS) and acts as an autocrine survival factor for tumor cell themselves. OS cell-specific aptamer (LC09) -functionalized PEG-PEI-Cholesterol (PPC) lipopolymer encapsulating CRISPR/Cas9 plasmids encoding VEGFA gRNA and Cas9 in both orthotopic OS and lung metastasis, showed effective VEGFA genome editing in tumor, decreased VEGFA expression and secretion, inhibited orthotopic OS malignancy and lung metastasis [98]. Zhang et al. evaluated G-protein-coupled Receptor Kinase Interactor-1(GIT1), as a target for the treatment of osteosarcoma and suggested that knowdown of GIT1 inhibited cell invasion and VEGF release in vitro and suppressed tumor growth, invasion, and angiogenesis in vivo, and also resulted in downregulation of hypoxia-inducible factor1α (HIF1α) and extracellular signal-regulated kinase (ERK1/2) pathways [99]. Moreover studies have shown that ALDH1B1, a subfamily of Aldehyde dehydrogenases (ALDHs), is upregulated in OS. Silencing of ALDH1B1 could inhibit the growth of xenograft tumor and knockdown of the same has shown to cause cycle arrest in G1 stage of OS cell in vitro cycle. Moreover, inhibition of ALDH1B1 expression could increase the sensitivity of chemotherapy [100]. The siRNA nanocarriers of chitosan-folic acid efficiently transferred the astrocyte elevated gene-1 (AEG-1) into the osteosarcoma cells, and knockdown of AEG-1 resulted in the inhibition of tumor cell proliferation and invasion [101].

11.5 Personalized nanomedicine for kidney disorders

The development of highly accurate biomarkers is essential for optimizing the management of kidney diseases. Various biomarkers of kidney diseases have been identified using proteomic techniques. Sequencing and genotyping can also help diagnose and treat kidney stones, cystic kidney disease, glomerulonephritis, and chronic kidney disorder. Besides, the pharmacogenomics predictors can help predict early-onset chronic kidney disease (CKD). Allelism in basement membrane–associated Fraser complex (FRAS1, FREM1, FREM2, GRIP1) is observed in CKD [102]. However, only a few of these biomarkers could be potentially used in clinical practice for development of personalized medicine. CKD273, has been validated and used in an interventional trial as a biomarker for early CKD detection, and has received a 'Letter-of-support' from the FDA [103].

The angiotensin-converting enzyme (ACE) gene encodes ACE, involved in the renin-angiotensin-aldosterone system and kinin–kallikrein pathway. ACE inhibitors are currently used in CKDs as renoprotective which reduce proteinuria and blood pressure. The genotyping approach is being used in patients with CKDs or transplantation, to treat patients who are nonresponsive to drugs. The polymorphism of Immunoglobulin Fc receptor (FcϒRIIIa) increases rituximab affinity by 10 folds and such polymorphisms may influence the efficacy of drugs. From transcriptome study on peripheral blood mononuclear cells (PBMCs) of uremic patients, the genes macrophage migration inhibitory factor, IL-8 receptor β and chemokine ligand 12 have been identified as potential therapeutic targets for reduction of inflammation in dialysis patients [104]. Gold (Au) and poly-actic-co-glycolic acid (PLGA) nanoparticles (NPs) loaded with fenoldopam (FD) targeted to dopamine-receptor type-5 (DR5) on primary cilia have been evaluated for the treatment of vascular hypertension in polycystic kidney disease (PKD) model through cilia targeting [105]. Podocytes play apivotal role in the progression of various kidney-related diseases. Vascular Cell Adhesion Molecule-1 (VCAM-1) expression is increased by podocytes upon TNFα-activation for upto 24 h and anti-VCAM-1 antibody can be employed as a ligand to facilitate the uptake of nanocarriers under inflammatory condition. Anti-VCAM-1-rapamycin-SAINT-O-Somes (lipid-based nanocarrier system) has been found to deliver the potent immunosuppressant rapamycin to TNFα-activated podocytes [106].

11.6 Personalized nanomedicine for gastrointestinal disorders

Functional gastrointestinal disorders (FGIDs) associated with impaired upper gastrointestinal (GI) due to delayed gastric emptying (GE), reduced gastric accommodation (GA), and functional lower GI symptoms including constipation-predominant irritable bowel syndrome, pelvic floor dyssynergia, colonic inertia, diarrhea-predominant irritable bowel syndrome, bile acid diarrhea, or act as a specific target for personalized medication. Hence, gastric relaxants or central neuromodulators, prokinetics are being used for personalized medicines in Functional Gastrointestinal Disorders (FGIDs). Personalized nanomedicine integrated with pharmacogenomics relates drug pharmacokinetics and drug enzymatic activity, specifically of CYP2D6, 2C19 and 3A4, to treat patients with FGIDs [107].

Orally delivered micellar nanoparticles, loaded with indomethacin developed by Yoshitomi et al., has potent nitroxide radical and ROS scavenging activity to treat small intestinal disorders [108]. Similarly, colon targeted hyaluronan-cisplatin

Drug Name	Nanoformulation	Indication	Phase*	References
DaunoXome/ Daunorubicin	Liposome	Acute myeloid leukemia, solid tumors, first-line treatment for patients with advanced HIV-associated Kaposi's sarcoma	Marketed	[114]
Genexol-PM/ Paclitaxel	PEG–PLA polymeric micelle	Breast, lung and ovarian cancer	Marketed	[115]
Abraxane/ Paclitaxel	Albumin nanoparticles	Metastatic Breast Cancer; Non-Small Cell Lung Cancer	Marketed	[116]
Doxil/Doxorubicin	PEGylated liposomes	Ovarian Cancer; Sarcoma; Myeloma	Marketed	[116]
Aroplatin/Cisplatin analog (L-NDDP)	Liposome	Malignant Mesothelioma	Phase II	[117]
DepoDur/ Morphine sulfate	Liposome	Pain management	Marketed	[118]
Invegasustenna/ Paliperidone palmitate	Nanocrystal	Schizophrenia	Marketed	[119]
Diprivan/Propofol	Nano-emulsion	Anesthetic	Marketed	[120]
siRNA transthyretin inhibitor	Lipid nanoparticles	Amyloidosis	Phase III	[121]
Tricor/Fenofibrate	Nanocrystal	Hypercholesterolemia	Marketed	[122]

*Note: PEG: poly (ethylene glycol); PLA: poly (lactic acid), PM: Polymeric miscelles, NSCLC: Non-small cell lung cancer, siRNA: Small interference RNA. *www.clinicaltrials.gov*

Table 5.
List of nanomedicines under clinical evaluation to target various diseases.

conjugated nanoparticles (HCNPs) has been developed by Tsai et al. for colon-specific drug delivery [109]. Also, CD98 siRNA/polyethyleneimine (PEI)-loaded NPs developed by Laroui et al. has shown down-regulation of intestinal CD98 for the treatment of colitis [110]. In addition, CS-TPP/IL-21 nanoparticles, Methotrexate loaded and folic acid conjugated guar gum nanoparticles (MTX-FA-GGNP), and deoxycholic acid conjugated nanoparticles (DexDA) loaded with retinoic acid have shown beneficial results in colorectal cancer [111–113].

Nonalcoholic fatty liver disease (NAFLD), including steatosis, fibrosis, and cirrhosis, leads to hepatocellular carcinoma. The CYP enzymatic activity that metabolizes different drugs can be affected by NAFLD. Hence, personalized treatment in all NAFLD patients is done through genetic profiling of the patient besides taking into account gender, environmental factors, diet habits, and CYP pattern to determine effective drug treatment. The polymeric nanoparticles such as the Smart Insulin L-490, a kind of personalized nanotheranostics, estimates patient glucose level and responds to the stimulus by releasing appropriate amount of insulin (**Table 5**) [123].

12. Future prospects

Regardless of contributions made by scientists, the adoption of pharmacogenetic testing in the clinical application has not been up to great extent [124]. The clinical trial of Tailor PCI study on the drug clopidogrel may increase the testing rates but presence of cheaper alternatives that does not require any pharmacogenetic testing may reverse the scenario [1]. Genome wide association studies which purport to give the well replicated data on genetic risk factors for complex diseases support the future of advanced application of pharmacogenetics. These novel risk factors may serve as potential therapeutic targets for the newly developed drugs and proper information about the patient genotype for these vital targets may affect the art of prescribing these drugs [125, 126]. Owing to these technology advanced settings, it is more likely that the pharmacogenetic knowledge will be available routinely in the near future, which will affect the science of prescribing drugs.

13. Conclusion

Pharmacogenomics is progressing in the form of personalized medicines in the world today. The main purpose of personalized therapies is to improve healthcare through the application of emerging technology. In these innovations, nanotechnology plays a key role with integration of pharmacogenomics to improve diagnosis and therapeutics at the individual level treatment. With this approach the introduction of personalized nanomedicine, has provided a major stimulus to the medicine and pharmacy disciplines to include advanced clinical therapies, disease management, diagnosis, and delivery of drugs.

Conflict of interest

The authors declare no conflict of interest.

Author details

Ruchi Chawla*, Varsha Rani, Mohini Mishra and Krishan Kumar
Department of Pharmaceutical Engineering and Technology, Indian Institute of Technology, Banaras Hindu University, Varanasi, Uttar Pradesh, India

*Address all correspondence to: rchawla.phe@iitbhu.ac.in

References

[1] Daly AK. Pharmacogenetics: A general review on progress to date [Internet]. Vol. 124, British Medical Bulletin. Oxford University Press; 2017 [cited 2020 Nov 17]. p. 65-79. Available from: https://academic.oup.com/bmb/article/124/1/65/4430783

[2] Roses AD. Pharmacogenetics. Hum Mol Genet. 2001 Oct;10(20):2261-2267.

[3] Pirmohamed M. Pharmacogenetics and pharmacogenomics [Internet]. Vol. 52, British Journal of Clinical Pharmacology. Wiley-Blackwell; 2001 [cited 2020 Nov 16]. p. 345-7. Available from: https://www.ncbi.nlm.nih.gov/pmc/articles/PMC2014592/

[4] Kalow W. Pharmacogenetics and pharmacogenomics: Origin, status, and the hope for personalized medicine. Vol. 6, Pharmacogenomics Journal. Pharmacogenomics J; 2006. p. 162-165.

[5] Zanger UM, Schwab M. Cytochrome P450 enzymes in drug metabolism: Regulation of gene expression, enzyme activities, and impact of genetic variation. Vol. 138, Pharmacology and Therapeutics. Pharmacol Ther; 2013. p. 103-141.

[6] Sim SC, Risinger C, Dahl ML, Aklillu E, Christensen M, Bertilsson L, Ingelman-Sundberg M. A common novel CYP2C19 gene variant causes ultrarapid drug metabolism relevant for the drug response to proton pump inhibitors and antidepressants. Clin Pharmacol Ther. 2006 Jan;79(1): 103-113.

[7] Johansson I, Lundqvist E, Bertilsson L, Dahl ML, Sjoqvist F, Ingelman- Sundberg M. Inherited amplification of an active gene in the cytochrome P450 CYP2D locus as a cause of ultrarapid metabolism of debrisoquine. Proc Natl Acad Sci U S A. 1993;90(24):11825-11829.

[8] Wang L, Weinshilboum R. Thiopurine S-methyltransferase pharmacogenetics: Insights, challenges and future directions. Vol. 25, Oncogene. Oncogene; 2006. p. 1629-1638.

[9] Tie JK, Stafford DW. Structural and functional insights into enzymes of the vitamin K cycle. Vol. 14, Journal of Thrombosis and Haemostasis. Blackwell Publishing Ltd; 2016. p. 236-247.

[10] The Cancer Genome Atlas Program - National Cancer Institute [Internet]. [cited 2021 Feb 1]. Available from: https://www.cancer.gov/about-nci/organization/ccg/research/structural-genomics/tcga

[11] Thorn CF, Klein TE, Altman RB. PharmGKB: The Pharmacogenomics Knowledge Base. [cited 2021 Feb 1]; Available from: www.pharmgkb.org,

[12] Relling M V, Krauss RM, Roden DM, Klein TE, Fowler DM, Terada N, Lin L, Riel-Mehan M, Do TP, Kubo M, Yee SW, Johnson GT, Giacomini KM, Pharmacol C, Author T. New Pharmacogenomics Research Network: An Open Community Catalyzing Research and Translation in Precision Medicine HHS Public Access Author manuscript. Clin Pharmacol Ther [Internet]. 2017 [cited 2021 Feb 1];102(6):897-902. Available from: http://www.pgrn.org/all-pgrn-publications.html

[13] Mestroni L, Begay R, Graw SL, Taylor MR. Pharmacogenetics of Heart Failure. [cited 2021 Feb 5]; Available from: http://www.genome.gov

[14] Limaye N. Pharmacogenomics, theranostics and personalized medicine - The complexities of clinical trials: Challenges in the developing world [Internet]. Vol. 2, Applied and Translational Genomics. Elsevier B.V.;

2013 [cited 2021 Feb 8]. p. 17-21. Available from: http://dx.doi.org/10.1016/j.atg.2013.05.002

[15] Sailani MR, Jahanbani F, Abbott CW, Lee H, Zia A, Rego S, Winkelmann J, Hopfner F, Khan TN, Katsanis N, Müller SH, Berg D, Lyman KM, Mychajliw C, Deuschl G, Bernstein JA, Kuhlenbäumer G, Snyder MP. Candidate variants in TUB are associated with familial tremor. Bućan M, editor. PLOS Genet [Internet]. 2020 Sep 21 [cited 2021 Feb 5];16(9):e1009010. Available from: https://dx.plos.org/10.1371/journal.pgen.1009010

[16] Truvé K, Parris TZ, Vizlin-Hodzic D, Salmela S, Berger E, Ågren H, Funa K. Identification of candidate genetic variants and altered protein expression in neural stem and mature neural cells support altered microtubule function to be an essential component in bipolar disorder. Transl Psychiatry [Internet]. 2020 Dec 1 [cited 2021 Feb 5];10(1):1-12. Available from: https://doi.org/10.1038/s41398-020-01056-1

[17] Cleynen I, Brants JR, Peeters K, Deckers R, Debiec-Rychter M, Sciot R, Van De Ven WJM, Petit MMR. HMGA2 Regulates Transcription of the Imp2 Gene via an Intronic Regulatory Element in Cooperation with Nuclear Factor-KB. Mol Cancer Res [Internet]. 2007 [cited 2021 Feb 9];5(4):363-72. Available from: http://www.genomatix.de

[18] Treutlein J, Kissling C, Frank J, Wiemann S, Dong L, Depner M, Saam C, Lascorz J, Soyka M, Preuss UW, Rujescu D, Skowronek MH, Rietschel M, Spanagel R, Heinz A, Laucht M, Mann K, Schumann G. Genetic association of the human corticotropin releasing hormone receptor 1 (CRHR1) with binge drinking and alcohol intake patterns in two independent samples. Mol Psychiatry [Internet]. 2006 Jun 21 [cited 2021 Feb 9];11(6):594-602. Available from: www.nature.com/mp

[19] Modena BD, Doroudchi A, Patel P, Sathish V. Leveraging genomics to uncover the genetic, environmental and age-related factors leading to asthma. In: Genomic and Precision Medicine: Infectious and Inflammatory Disease. Elsevier; 2019. p. 331-381.

[20] Zhang RZ, Pan TC, Zhang ZY, Mattei MG, Timpl R, Chu ML. Fibulin-2 (FBLN2): human cDNA sequence, mRNA expression, and mapping of the gene on human and mouse chromosomes. Genomics [Internet]. 1994 Jul 15 [cited 2021 Feb 9];22(2):425-30. Available from: http://www.ncbi.nlm.nih.gov/pubmed/7806230

[21] Paththinige CS, Sirisena ND, Dissanayake VHW. Genetic determinants of inherited susceptibility to hypercholesterolemia - a comprehensive literature review. Vol. 16, Lipids in Health and Disease. BioMed Central Ltd.; 2017.

[22] Kong Y, Xu K, Yuan K, Zhu J, Gu W, Liang L, Wang C. Digenetic inheritance of SLC12A3 and CLCNKB genes in a Chinese girl with Gitelman syndrome. BMC Pediatr [Internet]. 2019 Apr 18 [cited 2021 Feb 9];19(1). Available from: /pmc/articles/PMC6471809/

[23] Familial hypertrophic cardiomyopathy Precision Panel - Tests - GTR - NCBI [Internet]. [cited 2021 Feb 9]. Available from: https://www.ncbi.nlm.nih.gov/gtr/tests/514111/

[24] Lemaire SA, McDonald MLN, Guo DC, Russell L, Miller CC, Johnson RJ, Bekheirnia MR, Franco LM, Nguyen M, Pyeritz RE, Bavaria JE, Devereux R, Maslen C, Holmes KW, Eagle K, Body SC, Seidman C, Seidman JG, Isselbacher EM, Bray M, Coselli JS, Estrera AL, Safi HJ, Belmont JW, Leal SM, Milewicz DM. Genome-wide association study

identifies a susceptibility locus for thoracic aortic aneurysms and aortic dissections spanning FBN1 at 15q21.1. Nat Genet [Internet]. 2011 Oct [cited 2021 Feb 9];43(10):996-1002. Available from: /pmc/articles/PMC3244938/

[25] Behiry EG, Al-Azzouny MA, Sabry D, Behairy OG, Salem NE. Association of NKX2-5, GATA4, and TBX5 polymorphisms with congenital heart disease in Egyptian children. Mol Genet Genomic Med [Internet]. 2019 May 1 [cited 2021 Feb 9];7(5):612. Available from: /pmc/articles/PMC6503026/

[26] Hicks C, Pannuti A, Miele L. Associating GWAS information with the Notch signaling pathway using transcription profiling. Cancer Inform [Internet]. 2011 [cited 2021 Feb 9];10:93-108. Available from: /pmc/articles/PMC3091413/

[27] GWAS Catalog [Internet]. [cited 2021 Feb 9]. Available from: https://www.ebi.ac.uk/gwas/genes/NOTCH1

[28] cBioPortal for Cancer Genomics [Internet]. [cited 2021 Feb 8]. Available from: https://www.cbioportal.org/

[29] Cerami E, Gao J, Dogrusoz U, Gross BE, Sumer SO, Aksoy BA, Jacobsen A, Byrne CJ, Heuer ML, Larsson E, Antipin Y, Reva B, Goldberg AP, Sander C, Schultz N. The cBio Cancer Genomics Portal: An Open Platform for Exploring Multi dimensional Cancer Genomics Data: Figure 1. Cancer Discov [Internet]. 2012 May [cited 2021 Feb 8];2(5):401-4. Available from: http://cancerdiscovery.aacrjournals.org/lookup/doi/10.1158/2159-8290.CD-12-0095

[30] CellMiner - Analysis Tools [Internet]. [cited 2021 Feb 8]. Available from: https://discover.nci.nih.gov/cellminer/

[31] Reinhold WC, Sunshine M, Liu H, Varma S, Kohn KW, Morris J, Doroshow J, Pommier Y. CellMiner: A Web-Based Suite of Genomic and Pharmacologic Tools to Explore Transcript and Drug Patterns in the NCI-60 Cell Line Set. 2012 [cited 2021 Feb 8]; Available from: http://dtp.nci.nih.gov/

[32] [clue.io] [Internet]. [cited 2021 Feb 8]. Available from: https://clue.io/cmap

[33] Musa A, Ghoraie LS, Zhang SD, Glazko G, Yli-Harja O, Dehmer M, Haibe-Kains B, Emmert-Streib F. A review of connectivity map and computational approaches in pharmacogenomics. Brief Bioinform. 2018 May 1;19(3):506-523.

[34] MEDI and NDF-RT database developed by - Google Search [Internet]. [cited 2021 Feb 9].

[35] National Drug File - Reference Terminology - Summary | NCBO BioPortal [Internet]. [cited 2021 Feb 9]. Available from: https://bioportal.bioontology.org/ontologies/NDFRT

[36] SPHINX [Internet]. [cited 2021 Feb 9]. Available from: https://www.emergesphinx.org/

[37] Klein TE, Altman RB. PharmGKB: The pharmacogenetics and pharmacogenomics knowledge base [Internet]. Vol. 4, Pharmacogenomics Journal. Nature Publishing Group; 2004 [cited 2021 Feb 7]. p. 1. Available from: http://www.nature.com/tpj

[38] Thorn CF, Klein TE, Altman RB. PharmGKB: The pharmacogenomics knowledge base. Methods Mol Biol [Internet]. 2013 [cited 2021 Feb 7];1015:311-20. Available from: https://pubmed.ncbi.nlm.nih.gov/23824865/

[39] Sim SC, Ingelman-Sundberg M. The Human Cytochrome P450 (CYP) Allele Nomenclature website: A peer-reviewed database of CYP variants and their associated effects [Internet]. [cited 2021

Feb 7]. Available from: http://www.cypalleles.ki.se/

[40] Human Arylamine N-Acetyltransferase Gene Nomenclature — School of Medicine University of Louisville [Internet]. [cited 2021 Feb 7]. Available from: https://louisville.edu/medicine/departments/pharmacology/news-information/nat

[41] Ye AY, Liu Q-R, Li C-Y, Zhao M, Qu H. Human Transporter Database: Comprehensive Knowledge and Discovery Tools in the Human Transporter Genes. Xue Y, editor. PLoS One [Internet]. 2014 Feb 18 [cited 2021 Feb 7];9(2):e88883. Available from: https://dx.plos.org/10.1371/journal.pone.0088883

[42] Barbarino JM, Haidar CE, Klein TE, Altman RB. PharmGKB summary: very important pharmacogene information for UGT1A1. 2014 [cited 2021 Feb 7]; Available from: http://www.pharmacogenomics.pha.ulaval.ca/cms/ugt_alleles/

[43] Jain K. Role of nanobiotechnology in the development of personalized medicine. Nanomedicine [Internet]. 2009 Apr 30 [cited 2021 Feb 8];4(3):249-52. Available from: https://www.futuremedicine.com/doi/10.2217/nnm.09.12

[44] Bartlett G, Antoun J, Zgheib NK. Theranostics in primary care: Pharmacogenomics tests and beyond [Internet]. Vol. 12, Expert Review of Molecular Diagnostics. Taylor & Francis; 2012 [cited 2021 Feb 8]. p. 841-55. Available from: https://www.tandfonline.com/doi/abs/10.1586/erm.12.115

[45] Pharmacogenomics Technology (Theranostics & CDx) Market Worth $18.3 Billion By 2025: Grand View Research, Inc. [Internet]. [cited 2021 Feb 8]. Available from: https://www.prnewswire.com/news-releases/pharmacogenomics-technology-theranostics--cdx-market-worth-183-billion-by-2025-grand-view-research-inc-632846353.html

[46] Karachaliou N, Rosell R. Targeted treatment of mutated EGFR-expressing non-small-cell lung cancer: Focus on erlotinib with companion diagnostics [Internet]. Vol. 5, Lung Cancer: Targets and Therapy. Dove Medical Press Ltd.; 2014 [cited 2021 Feb 28]. p. 73-9. Available from: /pmc/articles/PMC5217512/

[47] Michaut M, Bader GD. Multiple genetic interaction experiments provide complementary information useful for gene function prediction. PLoS Comput Biol [Internet]. 2012 Jun [cited 2021 Feb 3];8(6). Available from: /pmc/articles/PMC3380825/?report=abstract

[48] Liu R, Zhao X, Liu X, Chen Z, Qiu L, Geng R, Guo W, He G, Yin J, Li J, Zhu & X. Influences of ERCC1, ERCC2, XRCC1, GSTP1, GSTT1, and MTHFR polymorphisms on clinical outcomes in gastric cancer patients treated with EOF chemotherapy.

[49] Weinshilboum R, Wang L. Pharmacogenomics: Precision Medicine and Drug Response. [cited 2021 Apr 3]; Available from: http://www.allelefrequencies.net/

[50] Van Allen EM, Miao D, Schilling B, Shukla SA, Blank C, Zimmer L, Sucker A, Hillen U, Foppen MHG, Goldinger SM, Utikal J, Hassel JC, Weide B, Kaehler KC, Loquai C, Mohr P, Gutzmer R, Dummer R, Gabriel S, Wu CJ, Schadendorf D, Garraway LA. Genomic correlates of response to CTLA-4 blockade in metastatic melanoma. Science (80-) [Internet]. 2015 Oct 9 [cited 2021 Feb 3];350(6257):207-11. Available from: https://pubmed.ncbi.nlm.nih.gov/26359337/

[51] Ciriello G, Miller ML, Aksoy BA, Senbabaoglu Y, Schultz N, Sander C.

Emerging landscape of oncogenic signatures across human cancers. Nat Genet [Internet]. 2013 Oct 26 [cited 2021 Feb 3];45(10):1127-33. Available from: https://www.nature.com/articles/ng.2762

[52] Amstutz U, Henricks LM, Offer SM, Barbarino J, Schellens JHM, Swen JJ, Klein TE, McLeod HL, Caudle KE, Diasio RB, Schwab M. Clinical Pharmacogenetics Implementation Consortium (CPIC) Guideline for Dihydropyrimidine Dehydrogenase Genotype and Fluoropyrimidine Dosing: 2017 Update. Clin Pharmacol Ther [Internet]. 2018 Feb 1 [cited 2021 Feb 9];103(2):210-6. Available from: http://doi.wiley.com/10.1002/cpt.911

[53] Plecko B, Steinfeld R. Disorders of Vitamin Metabolism. In: Swaiman's Pediatric Neurology: Principles and Practice: Sixth Edition. Elsevier Inc.; 2017. p. 373-82.

[54] Nguyen CM, Mendes MAS, Ma JD. Thiopurine methyltransferase (TPMT) genotyping to predict myelosuppression risk. PLoS Curr [Internet]. 2011 [cited 2021 Feb 9];3. Available from: /pmc/articles/PMC3094768/

[55] O'Dwyer PJ, Catalano RB. Uridine diphosphate glucuronosyltransferase (UGT) 1A1 and irinotecan: Practical pharmacogenomics arrives in cancer therapy. Vol. 24, Journal of Clinical Oncology. American Society of Clinical Oncology; 2006. p. 4534-8.

[56] Wang H, Gao X, Zhang X, Gong W, Peng Z, Wang B, Wang L, Chang S, Ma P, Wang S. Glutathione S-transferase gene polymorphisms are associated with an improved treatment response to cisplatin-based chemotherapy in patients with non-small cell lung cancer (NSCLC): A meta-analysis. Med Sci Monit [Internet]. 2018 Oct 20 [cited 2021 Feb 9];24:7482-92. Available from: /pmc/articles/PMC6204655/

[57] Haufroid V. Genetic Polymorphisms of ATP-Binding Cassette Transporters ABCB1 and ABCC2 and their Impact on Drug Disposition. Curr Drug Targets [Internet]. 2011 Apr 18 [cited 2021 Feb 9];12(5):631-46. Available from: https://pubmed.ncbi.nlm.nih.gov/21039333/

[58] Li Y, Liu F, Tan SQ, Wang Y, Li SW. X-Ray Repair Cross-Complementing Group 1 (XRCC1) Genetic Polymorphisms and Cervical Cancer Risk: A HuGE Systematic Review and Meta-Analysis. PLoS One [Internet]. 2012 Sep 12 [cited 2021 Feb 9];7(9). Available from: /pmc/articles/PMC3440401/

[59] Musunuru K, Roden DM, Boineau R, Bristow MR, McCaffrey TA, Newton-Cheh C, Paltoo DN, Rosenberg Y, Wohlgemuth JG, Zineh I, Hasan AAK. Cardiovascular pharmacogenomics: current status and future directions-report of a national heart, lung, and blood institute working group. J Am Heart Assoc [Internet]. 2012 Apr 12 [cited 2021 Feb 6];1(2):e000554. Available from: http://www.ncbi.nlm.nih.gov/pubmed/23130127

[60] Pereira NL, Keith Stewart MBChB A. Clinical Implementation of Cardiovascular Pharmacogenomics. 2015 [cited 2021 Feb 6]; Available from: http://dx.doi.org/10.1016/j.mayocp.2015.04.011

[61] Johnson JA, Cavallari LH. Pharmacogenetics and cardiovascular disease-implications for personalized medicine [Internet]. Vol. 65, Pharmacological Reviews. American Society for Pharmacology and Experimental Therapeutics; 2013 [cited 2021 Feb 4]. p. 987-1009. Available from: https://pharmrev.aspetjournals.org/content/65/3/987

[62] Zhu Y, Swanson KM, Rojas RL, Wang Z, St. Sauver JL, Visscher SL, Prokop LJ, Bielinski SJ, Wang L,

Weinshilboum R, Borah BJ. Systematic review of the evidence on the cost-effectiveness of pharmacogenomics-guided treatment for cardiovascular diseases [Internet]. Vol. 22, Genetics in Medicine. Springer Nature; 2020 [cited 2021 Feb 6]. p. 475-86. Available from: https://doi.org/10.1038/s41436-

[63] Roden DM, Van Driest SL, Wells QS, Mosley JD, Denny JC, Peterson JF. Opportunities and challenges in cardiovascular pharmacogenomics from discovery to implementation [Internet]. Vol. 122, Circulation Research. Lippincott Williams and Wilkins; 2018 [cited 2021 Feb 8]. p. 1176-90. Available from: http://circres.ahajournals.org

[64] Cacabelos R. Pharmacogenomic Biomarkers in Neuropsychiatry: The Path to Personalized Medicine in Mental Disorders.

[65] Vizirianakis IS, Miliotou AN, Mystridis GA, Andriotis EG, Andreadis II, Papadopoulou LC, Fatouros DG. Tackling pharmacological response heterogeneity by PBPK modeling to advance precision medicine productivity of nanotechnology and genomics therapeutics. Expert Rev Precis Med Drug Dev. 2019;4(3):139-151.

[66] Vizirianakis IS AE. Pharmaco genomics and nanotechnology toward advancing personalized medicine. In Springer, Berlin, Heidelberg; 2012. p. 115-34.

[67] Alharbi KK, Al-sheikh YA. Role and implications of nanodiagnostics in the changing trends of clinical diagnosis. Saudi J Biol Sci. 2014;21(2):109-117.

[68] Jhawat V, Gulia M, Gupta S, Maddiboyina B, Dutt R. Integration of pharmacogenomics and theranostics with nanotechnology as quality by design (QbD) approach for formulation development of novel dosage forms for effective drug therapy. J Control Release. 2020;327(August):500-511.

[69] Amstutz U, Carleton BC. Pharmacogenetic testing: Time for clinical practice guidelines. Clin Pharmacol Ther. 2011;89(6):924-927.

[70] Cheok MH, Lugthart S, Evans WE. Pharmacogenomics of acute leukemia. Annu Rev Pharmacol Toxicol. 2006;46:317-353.

[71] Gupta S, Jhawat V. Quality by design (QbD) approach of pharmacogenomics in drug designing and formulation development for optimization of drug delivery systems. Vol. 245, Journal of Controlled Release. Elsevier B.V.; 2017. p. 15-26.

[72] Eichelbaum M, Ingelman-Sundberg M, Evans WE. Pharmaco genomics and individualized drug therapy. Vol. 57, Annual Review of Medicine. 2006. p. 119-37.

[73] Mura S, Couvreur P. Nanotheranostics for personalized medicine. Adv Drug Deliv Rev. 2012;64(13):1394-1416.

[74] Wang LS, Chuang MC, Ho J an A. Nanotheranostics - A review of recent publications. Int J Nanomedicine. 2012;7:4679-4695.

[75] Rodríguez-Antona C, Taron M. Pharmacogenomic biomarkers for personalized cancer treatment. J Intern Med. 2015;277(2):201-217.

[76] Mäbert K, Cojoc M, Peitzsch C, Kurth I, Souchelnytskyi S, Dubrovska A. Cancer biomarker discovery: Current status and future perspectives. Int J Radiat Biol. 2014;90(8):659-677.

[77] Verma S, Prabhakar Y. Target Based Drug Design - A Reality in Virtual Sphere. Curr Med Chem. 2015;22(13):1603-1630.

[78] Cichonska A, Rousu J, Aittokallio T. Identification of drug candidates and repurposing opportunities through compound-target interaction networks. Expert Opin Drug Discov. 2015;10(12):1333-1345.

[79] Sharma S. Nanotheranostics in Evidence Based Personalized Medicine. Curr Drug Targets. 2020;15(10):915-930.

[80] Thurner GC, Chabicovsky M, Abdelmoez A, Debbage P. Targeted Drugs and Nanomedicine: Present and Future. Front Med Chem. 2016;182-233.

[81] Vizirianakis IS, Fatouros DG. Personalized nanomedicine: paving the way to the practical clinical utility of genomics and nanotechnology advancements. Vol. 64, Advanced Drug Delivery Reviews. 2012. p. 1359-62.

[82] Fruscella M, Ponzetto A, Crema A, Carloni G. The Extraordinary Progress in Very Early Cancer Diagnosis and Personalized Therapy: The Role of Oncomarkers and Nanotechnology. J Nanotechnol. 2016;2016.

[83] Jain KK. Role of nanobiotechnology in developing personalized medicine for cancer. Technol Cancer Res Treat. 2005;4(6):645-650.

[84] Atkinson SP, Andreu Z, Vicent MJ. Polymer therapeutics: Biomarkers and new approaches for personalized cancer treatment. J Pers Med. 2018;8(1).

[85] Choi, Y., Baker, J. R. J. Targeting Cancer Cells with DNA-Assembled Dendrimers. Cell Cycle. 2005;(May): 669-71.

[86] Schmieder AH, Winter PM, Caruthers SD, Harris TD, Williams TA, Allen JS, Lacy EK, Zhang H, Scott MJ, Hu G, Robertson JD, Wickline SA, Lanza GM. Molecular MR imaging of melanoma angiogenesis with α νβ3-targeted paramagnetic nanoparticles. Magn Reson Med. 2005;53(3):621-627.

[87] Gainkam LOT, Huang L, Caveliers V, Keyaerts M, Hernot S, Vaneycken I, Vanhove C, Revets H, De Baetselier P, Lahoutte T. Comparison of the biodistribution and tumor targeting of two 99mTc-labeled anti-EGFR nanobodies in mice, using pinhole SPECT/micro-CT. J Nucl Med. 2008;49(5):788-795.

[88] Cetin M, Gumru S, Aricioglu F. Nanotechnology applications in neuroscience: Advances, opportunities and challenges. Klin Psikofarmakol Bul. 2012;22(2):115-120.

[89] Kaushik A, Jayant RD, Bhardwaj V, Nair M. Personalized nanomedicine for CNS diseases. Drug Discov Today. 2018;23(5):1007-1015.

[90] Zheng M, Tao W, Zou Y, Farokhzad OC, Shi B. Nanotechnology-Based Strategies for siRNA Brain Delivery for Disease Therapy. Vol. 36, Trends in Biotechnology. Elsevier Ltd; 2018. p. 562-575.

[91] De Matteis L, Martín-Rapún R, de la Fuente JM. Nanotechnology in Personalized Medicine: A Promising Tool for Alzheimer's Disease Treatment. Curr Med Chem. 2017;25(35): 4602-4615.

[92] Kogan MJ, Bastus NG, Amigo R, Grillo-Bosch D, Araya E, Turiel A, Labarta A, Giralt E, Puntes VF. Nanoparticle-mediated local and remote manipulation of protein aggregation. Nano Lett. 2006;6(1):110-115.

[93] Zhao Y, J. Haney M. Active Targeted Macrophage-mediated Delivery of Catalase to Affected Brain Regions in Models of Parkinson?s Disease. Vol. 01, Journal of Nanomedicine & Nanotechnology. 2011.

[94] Buxton DB. Current status of nanotechnology approaches for cardiovascular disease: A personal perspective. Wiley Interdiscip Rev Nanomedicine Nanobiotechnology. 2009;1(2):149-155.

[95] Keyhanvar P, Bohlouli N, Bahrami S, Yousefzadeh A, Madadi S. Application of nanotechnology in device promotion in cardiology: A promising horizon for nanocardiology toward personalized medicine. Vol. 16, Iranian Heart Journal. 2015. p. 45-53.

[96] Li WF, Hou SX, Yu B, Jin D, Férec C, Chen JM. Genetics of osteoporosis: Perspectives for personalized medicine [Internet]. Vol. 7, Personalized Medicine. Per Med; 2010 [cited 2021 Apr 3]. p. 655-68. Available from: https://pubmed.ncbi.nlm.nih.gov/29788568/

[97] Cagnacci A, Venier M. The controversial history of hormone replacement therapy [Internet]. Vol. 55, Medicina (Lithuania). MDPI AG; 2019 [cited 2021 Apr 3]. Available from: /pmc/articles/PMC6780820/

[98] Liang C, Li F, Wang L, Zhang ZK, Wang C, He B, Li J, Chen Z, Shaikh AB, Liu J, Wu X, Peng S, Dang L, Guo B, He X, Au DWT, Lu C, Zhu H, Zhang BT, Lu A, Zhang G. Tumor cell-targeted delivery of CRISPR/Cas9 by aptamer-functionalized lipopolymer for therapeutic genome editing of VEGFA in osteosarcoma. Biomaterials. 2017 Dec 1;147:68-85.

[99] Zhang Z, Hu P, Xiong J, Wang S. Inhibiting GIT1 reduces the growth, invasionand angiogenesis of osteosarcoma. Cancer Manag Res [Internet]. 2018 [cited 2021 Apr 3];10:6445-55. Available from: /pmc/articles/PMC6278701/

[100] Wang X, Yu Y, He Y, Cai Q, Gao S, Yao W, Liu Z, Tian Z, Han Q, Wang W, Sun R, Luo Y, Li C. Upregulation of ALDH1B1 promotes tumor progression in osteosarcoma. Oncotarget [Internet]. 2018 [cited 2021 Apr 3];9(2):2502-14. Available from: /pmc/articles/PMC5788655/

[101] Wang F, Pang JD, Huang LL, Wang R, Li D, Sun K, Wang LT, Zhang LM. Nanoscale polysaccharide derivative as an AEG-1 siRNA carrier for effective osteosarcoma therapy. Int J Nanomedicine. 2018 Feb 8;13:857-875.

[102] Connaughton DM, Hildebrandt F. Personalized medicine in chronic kidney disease by detection of monogenic mutations. Nephrol Dial Transplant. 2020 Mar 1;35(3):390-397.

[103] Siwy J, Mischak H, Zürbig P. Proteomics and personalized medicine: a focus on kidney disease. Expert Rev Proteomics. 2019 Sep;16(9):773-782.

[104] Schena FP. Biomarkers and personalized therapy in chronic kidney diseases. Expert Opin Investig Drugs [Internet]. 2014 Aug 26 [cited 2021 Apr 3];23(8):1051-4. Available from: https://www.tandfonline.com/doi/full/10.1517/13543784.2014.922953

[105] Personalized nanomedicine for the treatment of vascular hypertension in polycystic kidney disease models – TechConnect Briefs [Internet]. [cited 2021 Apr 3]. Available from: https://briefs.techconnect.org/papers/personalized-nanomedicine-for-the-treatment-of-vascular-hypertension-in-polycystic-kidney-disease-models/

[106] K Visweswaran GRR, Gholizadeh S, RuitersMHJ, Molema G, Kok RJ, Kamps JAAM. Targeting Rapamycin to Podocytes Using a VascularCell Adhesion Molecule-1 (VCAM-1)-HarnessedSAINT-Based Lipid Carrier System. PLoS ONE. 2015; 10(9):e0138870. doi:10.1371/journal.pone.0138870

[107] Wang XJ, Camilleri M. Personalized medicine in functional gastrointestinal disorders: Understanding pathogenesis to increase diagnostic and treatment efficacy ORCID number: Conflict-of-interest statement. [cited 2021 Apr 4]; Available from: https://dx.doi.org/10.3748/wjg.v25.i10.1185

[108] Yoshitomi T, Sha S, Vong LB, Chonpathompikunlert P, Matsui H, Nagasaki Y. Indomethacin-loaded redox nanoparticles improve oral bioavailability of indomethacin and suppress its small intestinal inflammation. Ther Deliv [Internet]. 2014 Jan [cited 2021 Apr 4];5(1):29-38. Available from: https://pubmed.ncbi.nlm.nih.gov/24341815/

[109] Tsai SW, Yu DS, Tsao SW, Hsu FY. Hyaluronan-cisplatin conjugate nanoparticles embedded in eudragit S100-coated pectin/alginate microbeads for colon drug delivery. Int J Nanomedicine [Internet]. 2013 [cited 2021 Apr 4];8:2399-407. Available from: https://pubmed.ncbi.nlm.nih.gov/23861585/

[110] Laroui H, Geem D, Xiao B, Viennois E, Rakhya P, Denning T, Merlin D. Targeting intestinal inflammation with CD98 siRNA/PEI-loaded nanoparticles. Mol Ther [Internet]. 2014 [cited 2021 Apr 4];22(1):69-80. Available from: https://pubmed.ncbi.nlm.nih.gov/24025751/

[111] Xu Q, Guo L, Gu X, Zhang B, Hu X, Zhang J, Chen J, Wang Y, Chen C, Gao B, Kuang Y, Wang S. Prevention of colorectal cancer liver metastasis by exploiting liver immunity via chitosan-TPP/nanoparticles formulated with IL-12. Biomaterials [Internet]. 2012 May [cited 2021 Apr 4];33(15):3909-18. Available from: https://pubmed.ncbi.nlm.nih.gov/22374455/

[112] Sharma M, Malik R, Verma A, Dwivedi P, Banoth GS, Pandey N, Sarkar J, Mishra PR, Dwivedi AK. Folic acid conjugated guar gum nanoparticles for targeting methotrexate to colon cancer. J Biomed Nanotechnol [Internet]. 2013 Jan [cited 2021 Apr 4];9(1):96-106. Available from: https://pubmed.ncbi.nlm.nih.gov/23627072/

[113] Jeong Y Il, Chung KD, Kim DH, Kim YH, Lee YS, Choi KC. All-trans retinoic acid-incorporated nanoparticles of deoxycholic acid-conjugated dextran for treatment of CT26 colorectal carcinoma cells. Int J Nanomedicine [Internet]. 2013 Jan 29 [cited 2021 Apr 4];8:485-93. Available from: https://pubmed.ncbi.nlm.nih.gov/23390366/

[114] Eskandari Z, Bahadori F, Celik B, Onyuksel H. Targeted nanomedicines for cancer therapy, from basics to clinical trials. J Pharm Pharm Sci. 2020;23(1):132-157.

[115] Zhang Z, Mei L, Feng SS. Paclitaxel drug delivery systems. Expert Opin Drug Deliv. 2013;10(3):325-340.

[116] Zhong H, Chan G, Hu Y, Hu H, Ouyang D. A comprehensive map of FDA-approved pharmaceutical products. Pharmaceutics. 2018;10(4):1-19.

[117] Pooja D, Kadari A, Kulhari H, Sistla R. Lipid-based nanomedicines: Current clinical status and future perspectives. Lipid Nanocarriers for Drug Targeting. Elsevier Inc.; 2018. 509-528 p.

[118] Bulbake U, Doppalapudi S, Kommineni N, Khan W. Liposomal formulations in clinical use: An updated review. Pharmaceutics. 2017;9(2):1-33.

[119] Pandey A, Singh D, Dhas N, Tewari AK, Pathak K, Chatap V, Rathore KS, Mutalik *S. complex* injectables: Development, delivery, and advancement. Development, delivery, and advancement. Delivery of Drugs: Volume 2: Expectations and Realities of

Multifunctional Drug Delivery Systems. Elsevier Inc.; 2020. 191-213 p.

[120] Sarwal A, Singh G, Singh K, Garg S. Recent Interventions for Nanotechnology Based Drug Products: Insights into the Regulatory Aspects. Curr Pharm Des. 2019;24(43):5219-5228.

[121] Cullis PR, Hope MJ. Lipid Nanoparticle Systems for Enabling Gene Therapies. Mol Ther. 2017;25(7):1467-1475.

[122] Owuor JJ. Optimization and characterization of primaquine-loaded solid lipid nanoparticles (SLN) for liver schinonticide targeting by freeze drying. MOJ Drug Des Dev Ther. 2017;1(3):1-10.

[123] Fornaguera C, García-Celma MJ. Personalized nanomedicine: A revolution at the nanoscale [Internet]. Vol. 7, Journal of Personalized Medicine. MDPI AG; 2017 [cited 2021 Apr 4]. p. 12. Available from: www.mdpi.com/journal/jpm

[124] Cardon LR, Harris T. Precision medicine, genomics and drug discovery. Vol. 25, Human Molecular Genetics. Oxford University Press; 2016. p. R166–R172.

[125] Barrett JC, Dunham I, Birney E. Using human genetics to make new medicines. Vol. 16, Nature Reviews Genetics. Nature Publishing Group; 2015. p. 561-2.

[126] Nelson MR, Tipney H, Painter JL, Shen J, Nicoletti P, Shen Y, Floratos A, Sham PC, Li MJ, Wang J, Cardon LR, Whittaker JC, Sanseau P. The support of human genetic evidence for approved drug indications. Nat Genet. 2015 Aug;47(8):856-860.

Chapter 3

Interindividual Variability of Cytochromes P450 2B Mediated Oxidation in Human Liver

Abdulmohsen Alrohaimi, Bader Alrohaimi, Nada Alruwais and Kholoud Aldmasi

Abstract

The cytochromes P450 (CYPs) are a group of enzymes that are primarily responsible for oxidative drug biotransformation in people. CYP2B6, which metabolizes numerous drugs including bupropion, propofol and other drug shows great variability in rates of drug oxidation between individuals. In this chapter we discuss the contribution of selected genetic and environmental factors to this variability. Several studies identified and quantified the most common CYP2B6 mRNA splice such as deletion of exons 4 to 6 and of exon 4 which were significantly and negatively correlated with CYP2B6 protein and enzyme activity. CYP2B6 gene expression is highly inducible by phenobarbital. Alcohol ingestion has been associated with increased CYP2B6 levels this involves the constitutive androstane receptor (CAR) and/or the pregnane X receptor (PXR). CYP2B7 is considered a pseudogene because of the presence of a single premature stop codon (TGA) in exon 7. In 10 out of 24 African-Americans (but none out of 48 European-Americans) there is a single nucleotide polymorphism that results in an arginine codon instead of a stop codon (X378R). The results of these studies identify certain CYP2B6 genetic polymorphisms, mRNA splicing variants, and alcohol ingestion as significant factors that determine interindividual variability of CYP2B-mediated oxidation of drugs in people.

Keywords: Cytochromes, cytochromes P450, CYP2B6, CYP2B6 activity, drug oxidation

1. Introduction

Large interindividual variability in drug response is more of a rule than an exception. In fact, among patients treated with the same dose of drug, the response varies widely from no response at all to severe side effects. Many factors contribute to this variability, and apart from the role of non-pharmacological aspects, such as psychological and social issues, it mainly results from the interaction of genetic, pathophysiological and environmental factors that lead to interindividual differences in drug pharmacokinetics and pharmocodynamics. Since the discovery of the debrisoquine/sparteine hydroxylation polymorphism in 1970, research has expanded in the study of the interaction between environmental and genetic factors controlling the rate of drug metabolism. Currently, it is well known that cytochrome P450

(CYP) mediated drug metabolism shows large variability, leading to large differences in steady-state plasma concentrations of drugs. This variability is due to interaction of genetics and environmental factors. In addition, concomitant drug administration influences the variabilty of drug response. The main objective of the work described in this thesis dissertation was to study the role of genetic and environmental factors in determining interindividual variability of the CYP2B subfamily.

1.1 CYP enzymes

The cytochrome P450 (CYP) superfamily of enzymes plays a predominant role in the phase I metabolism of xenobiotics, environmental chemicals and endogenous compounds. An overview of the the most common reaction catalyzed by CYP is as follows:

$$R-H+O2+NADPH+H+\rightarrow R-OH+NADP++H2O \qquad (1)$$

The CYP enzymes are classified into families and subfamilies based on their amino acid sequence similarity. The CYP nomenclature is as follows: "P" stands for "pigment", "cyto" means "hollow vesicle", and "chrome" means "color". "450" is part of the name since the reduced enzyme absorbs light at 450 nm when bound to carbon monoxide. 'CYP' represents the CYP family. Members of the same family represented by a number (e.g. CYP2) share at least 40% identical with respect to their amino acid sequences. If the sequences are 40–55% identical, the enzymes belong to the same subfamily, indicated by an additional letter (e.g. CYP2B). Finally, each individual enzyme is represented by an Arabic numeral (e.g. CYP2B6). Three CYP gene families are mainly responsible for drug metabolism in humans and most other mammalian species i.e. CYP1, CYP2, and CYP3. CYP1 have two subfamilies CYP1A (i.e. CYP1A1 and 1A2) and CYP1B. CYP1A1 is mainly extrahepatic while CYP1A2 is a hepatic enzyme. Both are induced by polycyclic aromatic hydrocarbons (PAR), found for example in cigarette smoke and charbroiled meat. CYP1A2 is involved in metabolism of several. CYP2 is the largest family of human CYPs identified to date. In addition, there is 92% nucleotide sequence similarity of CYP2B7P with CYP2B6.

1.2 *In vitro* models used to study drug biotransformation

Various methods are used to study the metabolic activity of a CYP enzyme in vitro including human liver microsomes, recombinant expressed CYPs, cytosol, S9 fraction, cell lines, transgenic cell lines, primary hepatocytes, liver slices, and perfused liver.

1.2.1 Human liver microsomes

Human liver microsomes are prepared from fresh or frozen liver tissue, and contain different proportions of all CYPs for each donor. Human liver microsomes contain membrane bound Phase I enzymes and Phase II enzymes such as CYPs and UDP glucuronosyltransferases.

1.2.2 Recombinant CYPs

Individual CYPs (including 1A2, 2A6, 2B6, 2C8, 2C9, 2C19, 2D6, 2E1, 3A4, and 3A5) expressed in either lymphoblastoid cells or insect cells are available commercially from BD-Gentest Corporation [1].

1.2.3 Primary hepatocytes

Hepatocytes represent a model for studying biotransformation and drug–drug interactions, such as inhibition and induction [2]. One disadvantage of using hepatocytes is that availability is limited. Once a fresh liver is obtained, the hepatocytes must immediately be plated, used for suspension studies, or cryopreserved for future studies [2].

1.2.4 Liver slices

Liver slices represent one of the earliest in vitro models for metabolism studies, dating back to the earlier part of the 20th century [3].

1.2.5 S9 fraction

The S9 fraction is the fraction of the liver cellscontaining both microsomes and cytosol. It is obtained by centrigation of whole-liver homogenate at 9000 X g [4].

1.2.6 Liver cell lines

Liver cell lines are less popular compared to other models. This is mainly due to their dedifferentiated cellular characteristics and incomplete expression of all families of metabolic enzymes [5].

1.2.7 Bupropion hydroxylation as a CYP2B6 index reaction

If a substrate is biotransformed to one of its metabolites via only one CYP, the pathway is called an index reaction. In this thesis work, conversion of bupropion to hydroxybupropion was used as an index reaction for CYP2B6 based on the evidence as follows. Bupropion is biotransformed to three main metabolites in vivo, including hydroxybupropion, threohydrobupropion, and erythrohydrobupropion. Bupropion is biotransformed to the active metabolite hydroxybupropion mainly via CYP2B6 in vitro [6].

1.3 Factors influencing interindividual variability in CYP2B6 function

On average, CYP2B6 accounts for approximately 1 to 6% of total CYP450 [7, 8]. It was estimated that interindividual variability accounts for a 50-fold difference in CYP2B6 enzyme content [9]. Although CYP2B6 expression is highly variable, it is found at substantial levels in a small percentage of the population [6, 8, 10]. In addition, CYP2B6*6B haplotype and alcohol use history were identified as significant predictors of bupropion hydroxylation. The CYP2B6*6B haplotype was present at an allele frequency of 0.26. These correlations suggest that moderate alcohol consumption (at least 14 drinks of alcohol per week) is associated with enhanced CYP2B6 gene transcription, but the presence of at least one CYP2B6*6B allele reduces this inductive effect.

1.3.1 Genetic polymorphism

Genetic variation in CYPs may affect the biotransformation of drugs metabolized by those CYPs. Variation in a gene could arise from different causes. First, a single nucleotide polymorphism (SNP) is a single nucleotide variation in the genetic sequence. Another type of genetic variation is gene duplication in which a CYP gene is found in multiple copies.

1.3.2 *Effect of SNPs on CYP2B6* in vitro

Various laboratories have attempted to correlate CYP2B6 genotype with CYP2B6 phenotype in panels of human liver microsomes. Found novel point mutations in the CYP2B6 coding region: C64T, G516T, C777A, A785G and C1459T, at frequencies of 5.3%, 28.6%, 0.5%, 32.6% and 14.0%, respectively [11]. Furthermore, our laboratory has studied the correlation between several SNPs in the CYP2B6 coding and promoter region (to −3000 base pairs (bp)) verses bupropion hydroxylation activity, CYP2B6protein levels, and CYP2B6 mRNA levels *in vitro* were measured in a bank of 54 human livers.

Initial analysis showed excellent correlation between bupropion hydroxylation activities and CYP2B6 protein content (Rs = 0.88) but relatively poor correlation between CYP2B6 protein levels and CYP2B6 mRNA levels (Rs = 0.44) (**Figure 1A**). We did not find any individual genotypesthat significantly correlated with bupropion hydroxylation activity, CYP2B6 protein or mRNA levels, but found that alcohol use history and the CYP2B6*6B haplotype (−1456 t > c, −750 t > c, G516T, A785G [Q172H, K262R], p = 0.011) were significant predictors of bupropion hydroxylation (**Figure 1B**). The CYP2B6*6B haplotype was present at a frequency of 0.26 [10].

Jinno et al. [12] expressed CYP2B6 mutants (CYP2B6.2,.3,.4,.5,.6, and 7) in COS-1 cells and found that compared to wild type, CYP2B6.6 (G516T, A785G [Q172H, K262R]) was expressed at a lower protein level, but had significantly higher Km and Vmax values for activity of 7-ethoxy-4-trifluoromethylcoumarinO-deethylation (**Figure 1C**). Lang et al. identified four novel CYP2B6 alleles as phenotypic null alleles [13].

1.3.3 *Effect of SNPs* in vivo

When compared single-dose bupropion pharmacokinetics in 121 healthy male German Caucasian volunteers and found a correlation between the presence of the *4 allele (A785G [K262R]) and a higher (1.7-fold) bupropion clearance, although only a minor fraction of the variability in bupropion and hydroxybupropion kinetics could be explained by this variant [14]. Supporting our *in vitro* results, a clinical study involving efavirenz found that the CYP2B6*6 (G516T, A785G [Q172H, K262R]) genotype correlated with high plasma efavirenz concentrations in HIV-patients treated with standard efavirenz-containing regimens [15].

1.3.4 *Ethnic differences in CYP2B6 SNPs*

There are ethnic differences in the frequencies of CYP2B6 genotypes that could account for race/ethnic differences in CYP2B6 phenotype. For example, 89 Caucasians and 50 African-Americans who were receiving efavirenz treatment were genotyped for G516T [Q172H] [16].

1.3.5 *CYP2B6 inducers*

Various CYP2B6 inducers have been identified, including carbamazepine, phenobarbital and related barbiturates, and rifampin [17, 18].

1.4 Mechanisms of CYP induction

Post-transcriptional mechanisms include both mRNA and protein stabilization that may be mediated through transacting regulators or through changes in the phosphorylation status of the enzyme.

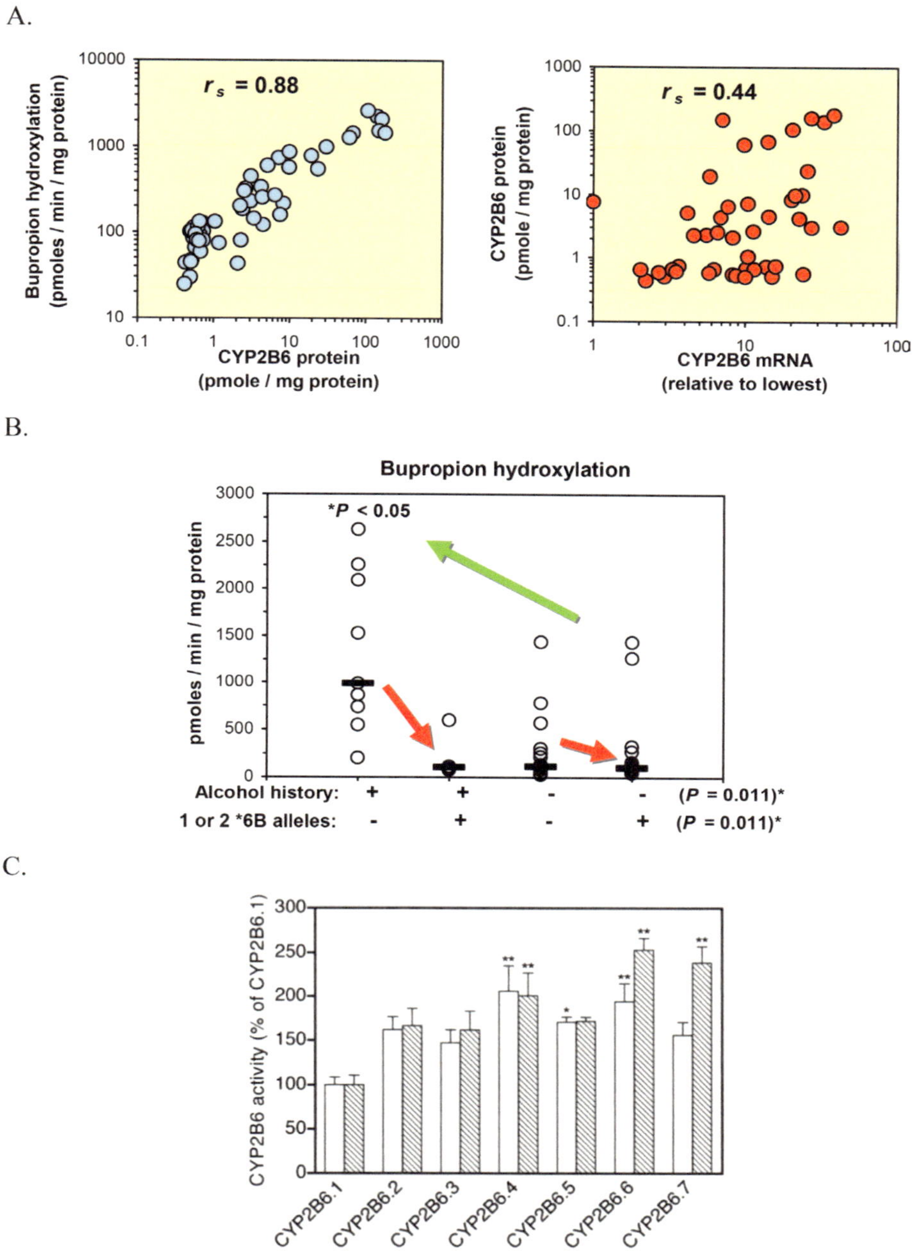

Figure 1.
*Data from our laboratory [10] showing relationships between CYP2B6 activities, protein content and mRNA content measured in a bank of 54 human livers (A); as well as effects of alcohol and *6B allele on CYP2B6 activity (B). A study by [12] showed that some CYP2B6 amino acid coding variants expressed in COS-1 cells are associated with higher activity (C).*

1.4.1 Transcriptional regulation

In addition to the induction of CYP1A genes, at least three other nuclear receptors (NRs) can induce transcription of drug metabolizing enzymes. These are the constitutive androstane receptor (CAR), the pregnane X receptor (PXR), and the peroxisome proliferator-activated receptor (PPAR).

1.4.2 Post-transcriptional regulation

Post-transcriptional regulation mechanisms include both mRNA and protein stabilization as well as stimulated of mRNA and protein degradation. These processes can result in an increase or decrease of enzyme expression, respectively. A good example is CYP2E1 that is regulated by several post-transcriptional mechanisms [19, 20].

1.5 Messenger RNA splicing

As seen in **Figure 2**, splicing is the process that results in excision of the introns from a pre-mRNA and the joining of the resultant exons. The splicing process is directed by special sequences at the intron/exon junctions called splice sites. The 5′ splice site marks the exon/intron junction at the 5′ end of the intron. This includes a GU dinucleotide at the intron end encompassed within a larger, less conserved consensus sequence. At the other end of theintron, the 3′ splice site region has three conserved sequence elements: the branch point, followed by a polypyrimidine tract, followed by a terminal AG at the extreme 3′ end of the intron. Splicing is carried out by the spliceosome, a large macromolecular complex that assembles onto these sequences and catalyzes the two transesterification steps of the splicing reaction. Splicing activators are generally thought to interact with components of the spliceosome to stabilize their binding to adjacent splice sites. SR (splicing regulator) proteins bind to exonic splicing enhancer elements or intronic enhancer elements to stimulate U2AF binding to the upstream 3⁻ splice site, or U1 snRNP binding to the downstream 5′ splice site (**Figure 2B**).

1.5.1 Alternative mRNA splicing

Alternative pre-mRNA splicing is a central mode of genetic regulation in higher eukaryotes (**Figure 3**). Alternative splicingplays an extremely important role in expanding protein diversityand might therefore partially explain the apparent

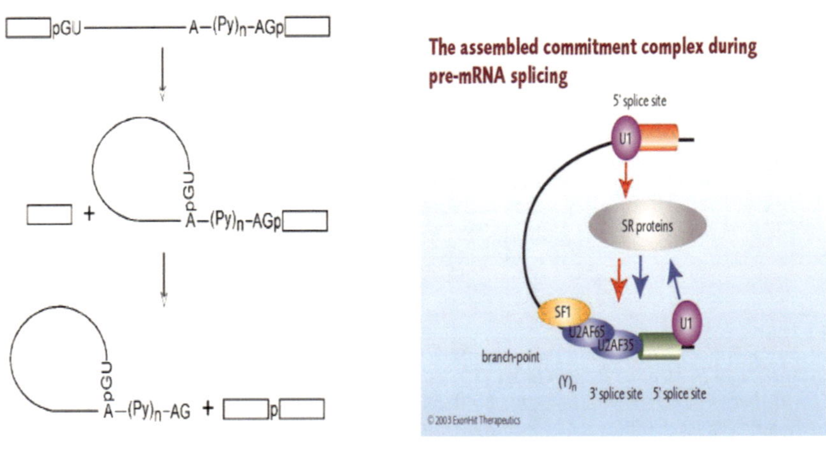

(A) (B)

Figure 2.
Molecular mechanisms involved in mRNA splicing. (A) Splicing takes place in two transesterification steps. The first step results in two reaction intermediates: the detached 5′- exon and an intron/3′-exon fragment in a lariat structure. The second step ligates the two exons and releases the intron lariat. (B) The complex can be converted into the active spliceosome and involves the recognition of the 5′ splice site by U1 snRNP and the branch-point sequence and 3′ splice site by SF1 and U2AF, respectively with the aid of SR proteins.

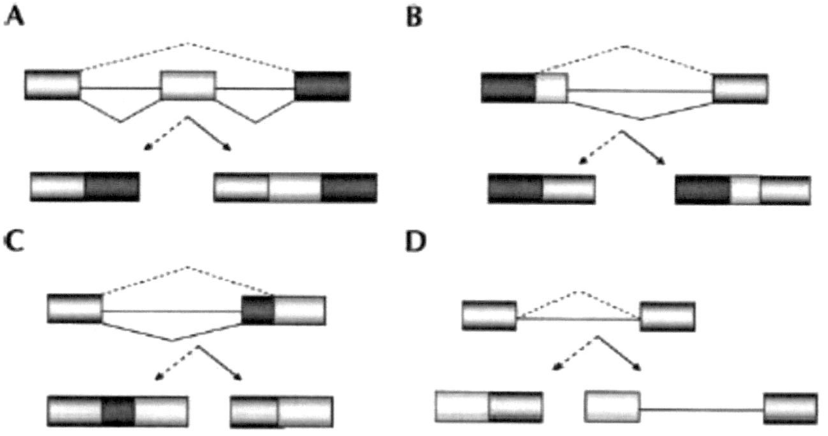

Figure 3.
Patterns of alternative splicing variation. Putative splice variants were classified according to the basic patterns of alternative splicing. (A) Cassette exon: an exon is spliced out with neighboring introns or included in the mature mRNA. (B) Internal donor site: competing donor (5′) splice sites exist for one acceptor site within an intron. (C) Internal acceptor site: competing acceptor (3′) splice sites exist for one donor site within an intron. (D) Retained intron: an intron is spliced out or included in RNA [20].

discrepancybetween gene number and organism complexity [21]. Approximately 40–60% of human genes are estimatedto have distinct splice variants [22]. The regulation of alternative splicing can involve on/off regulationof the products of particular genes and the production of alternativeproducts with clearly separable functions, often in a cell-type-specificmanner [23].

1.5.2 Regulation of splicing: SRproteins and regulatory elements

The SR proteins constitute the best-studied family of splicing regulators. The SR proteins have a common domain structure of one or two RNP-cs RNA binding domains followed by what is called an RS domain containing repeated arginine/serine dipeptides.

The RNA regulatory elements are enhancers or suppressors, diverse in sequence, and often embedded within nucleotides that also code for protein (exonic splice enhancers), but also found in introns. In the intron, the IEs and ISs are often found within a polypyrimidine tract or immediately adjacent to the branch point or 5′ splice site.

However, splicing regulatory elements can also act from a distance, being found hundreds of nucleotides away from the regulated exon.

SR proteins and exonic splicing enhancers (ESEs) play an important role in the regulation of alternative splicing. An SR protein binds to an ESE through its RNA-recognition motifs (RRM) and contacts the components of a spliceosome through its RS domain. Errors in splicing regulation have been implicated in a number of different disease states.

1.6 Effect of alcohol on CYP genes

A Chronic exposure to alcohol produces change in gene expression and alcoholics suffer long-term dysfunction in multiple organ systems, including the liver, immune system and heart [24]. Alcohol is likely to be involved in a significant number of adverse drug reactions.

1.6.1 *Inductive effects of ethanol* in vitro

Alcohol has been shown to induce hepatic drug metabolism [25].

If administered after a chronic period of alcohol consumption, drugs that are metabolized by enzymes induced by alcohol may have significantly altered biotransformation.

It is found that incubation with ethanol and isopentanol resulted in a synergistic induction of CYP2B1/2 activity and protein levels in cultured rat hepatocytes; and an additive to synergistic induction of CYP2H1/2 activity and protein levels in cultured chick hepatocytes [26].

1.6.2 *Inductive effects of ethanol in animals* in vivo

It is well established that CYP2E1 is induced by alcohol in humans. In vitro and in vivo human clinical studies have shown that CYP2E1 is induced by ethanol [27–29]. The metabolic ratio of CYP2E1 activity was higher in a group of volunteers that were drinking at least 80 grams of ethanol per day for at least 5 years compared to abstaining alcoholics (for 14 days) and nonalcoholics with liver disease.

In a study subjects drank 40 grams of red wine for a total of four weeks and the metabolic ratio of CYP2E1 activity increased starting after one week of drinking, indicating increased CYP2E1 activity [28]. The ratio continuously increased when measured each week throughout the four-week study.

Brain samples from smoking alcoholics compared to nonsmoking, nondrinking subjects showed increased CYP2B6 protein expression as determined by western blot analysis. In Chapter 3 we use human hepatic and intestinal cell lines to determine whether ethanol can induce CYP2B6 and CYP2B7 mRNA expression; and also explore a role for the nuclear receptor CAR and/or PXR in this induction.

1.6.3 *Inhibiting effects of ethanol* in vitro

In vitro, concentrations of ethanol (0.1–3%) had inhibitory effects on CYPs 1A1, 1A2, 2A6, 2B6, 2C8, 2C19, 2D6, and 3A4. In human liver microsomes, ethanol inhibits the biotransformation of CYP3A substrates nifedipine, triazolam, and testosterone [30].

1.6.4 *Inhibiting effects of ethanol* in vivo

There is evidence that an acute dose of alcohol inhibits some human CYPs in vivo. In vitro data may explain the observations that acute ethanol intoxication potentiates the action of barbiturates, while there is increased resistance to the action of some sedatives in sober alcoholics. Ethanol does not appear to inhibit CYP2B6 in vivo in humans since it did not alter pharmacokinetics of bupropion when acutely coadministered with bupropion [31].

1.7 CYP pseudogenes

Pseudogenes are disabled copies of genes that do not produce a functional, full-length copy of a protein. They are of two main types of pseudogenes. Firstly, there are processed pseudogenes. Secondly, there are nonprocessed pseudogenes [32, 33]. With subsequent evolutionary time (generations), these pseudogenes accumulate further coding and noncoding disablements. There are other types of protein-related pseudogenes that are not accounted for in the above classification including semiprocessed pseudogenes.

The extent of the pseudogene population in the human genome is not yet clear. It has been estimated that thereare ~9000 processed and ~ 10,000 nonprocessed pseudogenesin the human genome; [34, 35]. A review of available genomic information indicates that there are many pseudogenes in the CYP family, and it has estimated that there may be more CYP pseudogenes than functional genes within the drug metabolizing enzyme families – CYP 1, 2 and 3 (see **Table 1**). A focus of the studies described in Chapter 4 of this dissertation is CYP2B7P. CYP2B7P has been identified as a pseudogene due to the presence of a single nucleotide change resulting in a premature stop codon in exon 7 (X378) and predicted truncated protein [36].

CYPs	Function	Genes/pseudogenes
CYP1	drug metabolism	(3 subfamilies 3 genes 1 pseudogene).
CYP2	drug and steroid metabolism	(13 subfamilies 16 genes 16 pseudogenes).
CYP3	drug metabolism	(1 subfamily 4 genes 2 pseudogenes).
CYP4	arachidonic acid or fatty acid metabolism	(5 subfamilies 11 genes 10 pseudogenes).
CYP5	thromboxane A2 synthase	(1 subfamily 1gene).
CYP7A	bile acid biosynthesis 7-alpha hydroxylase of steroid nucleus	(1 subfamily member).
CYP7B	brain specific form of 7-alpha hydroxylase	(1 subfamily member)
CYP8A	prostacyclin synthase	(1 subfamily member).
CYP8B	bile acid biosynthesis	(1 subfamily member).
CYP11	steroid biosynthesis	(2 subfamilies 3 genes).
CYP17	steroid biosynthesis 17-alpha hydroxylase	(1 subfamily 1 gene).
CYP19	steroid biosynthesis aromatase forms estrogen	(1 subfamily 1 gene).
CYP20	Unknown function	(1 subfamily 1 gene).
CYP21	steroid biosynthesis	(1 subfamily 1 gene 1 pseudogene).
CYP24	vitamin D degradation	(1 subfamily 1 gene).
CYP26A	retinoic acid hydroxylase	(1 subfamily member).
CYP26B	probable retinoic acid hydroxylase	(1 subfamily member).
CYP26C	probabvle retinoic acid hydroxylase	(1 subfamily member).
CYP27A	bile acid biosynthesis	(1 subfamily member).
CYP27B	vitamin D3 1-alpha hydroxylase activates vitamin D3 (1 subfamily member).	
CYP27C	unknown function	(1 subfamily member).
CYP39	7 alpha hydroxylation of 24 hydroxy cholesterol	(1 subfamily member).
CYP46	cholesterol 24-hydroxylase	(1 subfamily member).
CYP51	cholesterol biosynthesis lanosterol 14-alpha demethylase	(1 subfamily 1 gene 3 pseudogenes).

Table 1.
Human CYP genes and pseudogenes.

In Chapter 4 we determine whether CYP2B7P is a polymorphic gene in humans, and whether there are genetic variants that code for a full length CYP2B7 protein, lacking the common stop codon (X378). We also evaluate whether the recombinant full-length variant CYP2B7 (R378) is capable of hydroxylating the CYP2B6 substrate bupropion.

2. Conclusion

The main objective of the work described in this thesis dissertation was to study the role of genetic and environmental factors in determining interindividual variability of the CYP2B subfamily.

The results of these studies identify certain CYP2B6 genetic polymorphisms, mRNA splicing variants, and alcohol ingestion as significant factors that determine interindividual variability of CYP2B-mediated oxidation of drugs in people.

Acknowledgements

Indeed, this work would not have been come to pass without the aid and encouragement of so many people. Actually, this piece of work has been a collective effort and by no means my sole product. Family and friends are at the core of this accomplishment, constantly providing us with encouraging words to get through tougher times. So, we greatly acknowledge the contribution of the sincere people who so graciously supported us throughout this work which would not have been accomplished without the support and assistance of them, so we are really grateful and ask Allah to reward them on our behalf.

Author details

Abdulmohsen Alrohaimi[1*], Bader Alrohaimi[2], Nada Alruwais[1] and Kholoud Aldmasi[1]

1 Shaqra University, Riyadh, Saudi Arabia

2 King Saud bin Abdulaziz University for Health Sciences, Riyadh, Saudi Arabia

*Address all correspondence to: alrohaimi@su.edu.sa

References

[1] NOTLEY LM, WOLF, C. J F., WUNSCH, R. M., ROY G LANCASTER, R. G. Bioactivation of Tamoxifen by Recombinant Human Cytochrome P450 Enzymes. Chemical Research in Toxicology. 2002;**15**(5):614-622

[2] LI, A. P., REITH, M. K., RASMUSSEN, A., GORSKI, J. C., HALL, S. D., XU, L., KAMINSKI, D. L. & CHENG, L. K. Primary human hepatocytes as a tool for the evaluation of structure-activity relationship in cytochrome P450 induction potential of xenobiotics: evaluation of rifampin, rifapentine and rifabutin. Chem Biol Interact. 1997;**107**:17-30

[3] EKINS S, RING BJ, GRACE J, MCROBIE-BELLE DJ, WRIGHTON SA. Present and future in vitro approaches for drug metabolism. J Pharmacol Toxicol Methods. 2000;**44**:313-324

[4] RICHARDSON, S. J., BAI, A., KULKARNI A. A, AND MOGHADDAM, M. F. (2016) Efficiency in Drug Discovery: Liver S9 Fraction Assay As a Screen for Metabolic Stability. Drug Metabolism Letters. 10(2): 83-90

[5] SUEYOSHI T, KAWAMOTO T, ZELKO I, HONKAKOSKI P, NEGISHI M. The repressed nuclear receptor CAR responds to phenobarbital in activating the human CYP2B6 gene. J Biol Chem. 1999;**274**:6043-6046

[6] HESSE LM, VENKATAKRISHNAN K, COURT MH, VON MOLTKE LL, DUAN SX, SHADER RI, et al. CYP2B6 mediates the In vitro hydroxylation of bupropion: potential drug interactions with other antidepressants. Drug Metabolism and Disposition. 2000;**28**: 1176-1183

[7] SHIMADA T, YAMAZAKI H, MIMURA M, INUI Y, GUENGERICH F. Interindividual variations in human liver cytochrome P-450 enzymes involved in the oxidation of drugs, carcinogens and toxic chemicals: Studies with liver microsomes of 30 Japanese and 30 caucasians. The Journal of Pharmacology and Experimental Therapeutics. 1994;**270**:414-423

[8] STRESSER D, KUPFER D. Monospecific antipeptide antibody to cytochrome P-450 2B6. Drug Metabolism and Disposition. 1999;**27**: 517-525

[9] TRACY TS, CHAUDHRY AS, PRASAD B, THUMMEL KE, SCHUETZ EG, ZHONG X, et al. Interindividual Variability in Cytochrome P450–Mediated Drug Metabolism. Drug Metabolism Disposition. 2016;**44**(3): 343-351

[10] HESSE LM, HE, P., KRISHNASWAMY, S., HAO, Q., HOGAN, K., VON MOLTKE, L. L., GREENBLATT, D. J. & COURT, M. H. Pharmacogenetic determinants of interindividual variability in bupropion hydroxylation by cytochrome P450 2B6 in human liver microsomes. Pharmacogenetics. 2004;**14**:225-238

[11] LANG T, KLEIN K, FISCHER J, NUSSLER AK, NEUHAUS P, HOFMANN U, et al. Extensive genetic polymorphism in the human CYP2B6 gene with impact on expression and function in human liver. Pharmacogenetics. 2001;**11**:399-415

[12] JINNO H, TANAKA-KAGAWA T, OHNO A, MAKINO Y, MATSUSHIMA E, HANIOKA N, et al. Functional characterization of cytochrome P450 2B6 allelic variants. Drug MetabDispos. 2003;**31**:398-403

[13] LANG T, KLEIN K, RICHTER T, ZIBAT A, KERB R, EICHELBAUM M, et al. Multiple novel nonsynonymous CYP2B6 gene polymorphisms in

Caucasians: demonstration of phenotypic null alleles. J Pharmacol-ExpTher. 2004;**311**:34-43

[14] KIRCHHEINER J, KLEIN C, MEINEKE I, SASSE J, ZANGER UM, MURDTER TE, et al. Bupropion and 4-OH-bupropion pharmacokinetics in relation to genetic polymorphisms in CYP2B6. Pharmacogenetics. 2003;**13**: 619-626

[15] TSUCHIYA K, GATANAGA H, TACHIKAWA N, TERUYA K, KIKUCHI Y, YOSHINO M, et al. Homozygous CYP2B6 *6 (Q172H and K262R) correlates with high plasma efavirenz concentrations in HIV-1 patients treated with standard efavirenz-containing regimens. Biochem Biophys Res Commun. 2004;**319**:1322-1326

[16] HAAS DW, RIBAUDO HJ, KIM RB, TIERNEY C, WILKINSON GR, GULICK RM, et al. Pharmacogenetics of efavirenz and central nervous system side effects: an Adult AIDS Clinical Trials Group study. Aids. 2004;**18**: 2391-2400

[17] PASCUSSI JM, BUSSON-LE CONIAT, M., MAUREL, P. & VILAREM, M. J. Transcriptional analysis of the orphan nuclear receptor constitutive androstane receptor (NR1I3) gene promoter: identification of a distal glucocorticoid response element. Mol Endocrinol. 2003;**17**:42-55

[18] DROCOURT L, OURLIN JC, PASCUSSI JM, MAUREL P, VILAREM MJ. Expression of CYP3A4, CYP2B6, and CYP2C9 is regulated by the vitamin D receptor pathway in primary human hepatocytes. J Biol Chem. 2002;**277**: 25125-25132

[19] BEVILACQUA A, CERIANI MC, CAPACCIOLI S, NICOLIN A. Post-Transcriptional Regulation of Gene Expression by Degradation of Messenger RNAs. Journal of cellular physiology. 2003;**195**:356-372

[20] FRANKS A, AIROLDI E, SLAVOV N. Post-transcriptional regulation across human tissues. PLOS Computational Biology, l. 2017;**13**(5)

[21] GRAVELEY, B. R. (2001). Alternative Splicing: Increasing Diversity in the Proteomic World. Trends in Genetics, 17(2):100-107

[22] LEE, C. AND ROY, M. (2004) Analysis of alternative splicing with microarrays: successes and challenges. Genome Biol., 5(7): 231

[23] WANG Y, LIU J, HUANG B, XU, Y., LI, J., HUANG, L., LIN, J., ZHANG, J., MIN, Q., YANG, W., and WANG, X. Mechanism of alternative splicing and its regulation. Biomedical Reports. 2015;**3**(2):152-158

[24] DGUZEH U, HADDAD NC, SMITH KT, JOHNSON JO, DOYE AA, GWATHMEY, J. K AND HADDAD G. E. Alcoholism: A Multi-Systemic Cellular Insult to Organs. Int J Environmental Research and Public Health. 2018;**15**(6): 1083

[25] JIN, M., ANDE, A., KUMAR, A. AND KUMAR, S. (2013) Regulation of cytochrome P450 2e1 expression by ethanol: role of oxidative stress-mediated pkc/jnk/sp1 pathway. Cell Death & Disease, 4: e554

[26] LOUIS CA, SINCLAIR JF, WOOD SG, LAMBRECHT LK, SINCLAIR PR, SMITH EL. Synergistic induction of cytochrome P450 by ethanol and isopentanol in cultures of chick embryo and rat hepatocytes. Toxicology and Applied Pharmacology. 1993;**118**(2): 169-176

[27] YE Q.,, LIAN, F., CHAVEZ, P. R., CHUNG, J., LING, W., QIN, H., SEITZ, H. K., and WANG, X. (2012) Cytochrome P450 2E1 inhibition prevents hepatic carcinogenesis induced by diethylnitrosamine in alcohol-fed rats. Hepatobiliary Surgury and Nutrition, 1(1): 5-18.

[28] ONETA CM, LIEBER CS, LI, J., RUTTIMANN, S., SCHMID, B., LATTMANN, J., ROSMAN, A. S. & SEITZ, H. K. Dynamics of cytochrome P4502E1 activity in man: induction by ethanol and disappearance during withdrawal phase. J Hepatol. 2002; **36**:47-52

[29] RAUCY JL, LASKER J, OZAKI K, ZOLETA V. Regulation of CYP2E1 by ethanol and palmitic acid and CYP4A11 by clofibrate in primary cultures of human hepatocytes. Toxicol Sci. 2004; **79**:233-241

[30] PENG Y, WU, H., ZHANG, X., ZHANG, F. A comprehensive assay for nine major cytochrome P450 enzymes activities with 16 probe reactions on human liver microsomes by a single LC/MS/MS run to support reliable in vitro inhibitory drug–drug interaction evaluation. Xenobiotica. 2015;**45**(11): 1-17

[31] POSNER J, BYE A, JEAL S, PECK AW, WHITEMAN P. Alcohol and bupropion pharmacokinetics in healthy male volunteers. Eur J ClinPharmacol. 1984;**26**:627-630

[32] MIGHELL, A.J., SMITH N.R., ROBINSON P.A. & MARKHAM A.F. (2000) Vertebrate pseudogenes. *FEBS Lett*468, 109-114.

[33] VANIN, E. F. (1985) Processed pseudogenes: characteristics and evolution. Annu Rev Genet, 19, 253-272.

[34] TUTAR, Y. (2012) Pseudogenes. Comparative and Functional Genomics: 4

[35] ZHANG Z, HARRISON PM, LIU Y, AND GERSTEIN, M. Millions of Years of Evolution Preserved: A Comprehensive Catalog of the Processed Pseudogenes in the Human Genome. Genome Research. 2003; **13**(12):2541-2558

[36] ZANGER, U. M. AND SCHWAB, M. (2013) Cytochrome P450 enzymes in drug metabolism: Regulation of gene expression, enzyme activities, and impact of genetic variation. Pharmacology & Therapeutics, Volume 138, Issue 1: 103-141

Chapter 4

Ivan Illich, Iatrogenesis and Pharmacogenetics

José Antonio Diniz de Oliveira

Abstract

In Medical Nemesis - The expropriation of health, IVAN ILLICH highlights several aspects of the medicalization of society, which was already observed in the mid-1970s. He addressed the various forms of iatrogenesis, classifying the new disease caused by the set of medical care as an epidemic that would not exist if there were no medical intervention. Of the various forms of iatrogenesis, he also addressed drug iatrogenesis, including the cause of hospital admissions. In this article, more than 40 years after Illich's seminal publication, we sought to revisit his thinking and assess the relevance of his narrative regarding the inconveniences resulting from the use of medicines, especially in their impacts on hospitalization, in addition to reflecting on the potential of pharmacogenetics to mitigate adverse events related to drugs that victimize people. After a brief presentation of Illich's trajectory, a digression is made on the association between the concepts of medicalization and iatrogenesis, to then make quick considerations about social iatrogenesis, considering the effects of this phenomenon on society. After presenting the consequences of iatrogenesis, from a fluent literature review, an update of the findings is made, showing that the problem is relevant today. A brief conceptual presentation of pharmacogenetics is followed by some examples of its clinical consequences. It is concluded that, despite the unequivocal importance of pharmacotherapy, iatrogenesis remains a problem of increasing relevance. Pharmacogenetics presents itself as a possibility to minimize the problem, making it possible to expand its use in the practice of medical services.

Keywords: Medicalization, iatrogenic disease, adverse effects, pharmacogenetics

1. Introduction

> *"Almost all men die from their drugs and not from their diseases"*
> *(Molière - 1622-1673, The Imaginary Invalid, Act III).*

In his work devoted to analyzing the theme of health, Ivan Illich addressed the medicalization of society, the harms caused by the medical apparatus, the so-called iatrogenesis, including drug iatrogenesis, which he also listed as the cause of hospital admissions [1].

Revisited more than 40 years after its publication, the work 'Medical Nemesis' still proves to be thought provoking and current. More than stimulating reflection, it has the strength to motivate the investigation of several of the aspects it addresses, so that one can know, for example, whether iatrogeneses related to hospital admissions are still a public health problem, a topic that has been extensively discussed. Extensive investigation [2–4].

Although adverse drug events (ADE) often include errors that occurred before and during hospitalization, even the correct prescriptions can present iatrogenesis, a situation that occurs when they cause more harm than good. In addition to the direct losses to patients, ADEs influence to increase the already unsustainable costs of health systems.

Therefore, iatrogenesis is not just a result of an error in the prescription. It is relatively common to have a correct diagnosis and prescription, but undesirable results due to several aspects. One of them has the explanation for the adverse effect in genetics. The literature also refers to writing iatrogenesis, when difficult to read writing causes potential or real problems to patients [5].

On the other hand, the contribution of drugs towards the cure or control of various diseases is undisputed, with a direct impact on prolongation and quality of life.

The association between drugs and different responses to treatments explained by individuals' genetic variants is an ancient discovery, confirmed by several scientists since the beginning of the last century [6]. The knowledge arising from the human genome project has led to advances in several fields of modern science, but it is in the field of Health, in particular, that its applicability has been growing in a promising way [7].

In Health, the discoveries of genomics have contributed to improve the assertiveness of diagnoses, prognoses and treatments, including those related to the ingestion of medications, which makes pharmacogenetics one of the main manifestations of the so-called precision medicine.

It may sound inconsistent to relate Ivan Illich - an iconoclast of health technologies and an opponent of everything that stimulates the medicalization of society - with pharmacogenetics, after all, one of the most advanced technologies. However, this new branch of science, which constitutes one of the most promising forms of the applicability of genomic findings, can respond to an important problem highlighted by the author (adverse drug reaction) that causes discomfort in people and increases the already unsustainable costs of the health system, especially when such effects result in hospital admissions [8].

The purpose of this article is to revisit Ivan Illich's thinking and discuss the currentness of his complaints regarding the inconveniences arising from the use of drugs, especially in their impact on hospitalization, and also reflect on the potential of pharmacogenetics to mitigate adverse events related to drugs that victimize people.

In the text that follows, it begins with a brief presentation of Illich's story. Thereafter, a digression is made on the association between the concepts of medicalization and iatrogenesis, to then make quick considerations about social iatrogenesis, considering the effects of this phenomenon on society. After presenting the consequences of iatrogenesis as proposed by Illich, from a fluent literature review, an update of the findings is made, providing evidence that the problem shows to be current and relevant nowadays. A quick conceptual presentation of pharmacogenetics is followed by examples of its clinical consequences in specific pharmacological groups.

2. About Ivan Illich and medicalization

Born in Austria in 1926, Ivan Illich is the owner of an extraordinary life trajectory. He resided in Florence, Italy, where he studied Natural Sciences with a specialization in inorganic chemistry and crystallography. In Rome, he graduated in Philosophy and Theology, and was ordained a priest. Subsequently, he completed a doctoral degree in Medieval History at the University of Salzburg [9], Austria, and a post-doctoral degree at the Princeton University, USA. At the Vatican, he would be used in diplomatic functions, but in 1951 he preferred to be a parish priest in New York, USA. The parish served the Puerto Rican community, which led him to occupy, in 1956, the vice-rectory at the Catholic University of Puerto Rico [10]. He traveled alone through South America and in 1961 created, in Cuernavaca, in Mexico, a center for studies and preparation of missionaries for Latin America. Finally, in Bremen, Germany, he was a visiting professor - as, indeed, at several world-renowned universities - and died on December 2, 2002 [11]. Due to the plurality of themes that he studied, explained in greater detail and which he published on, he was considered a polymath - "an individual who knows a lot, who studies or who knows many sciences", in addition to polyglot, having mastered 10 different languages [9].

He was a controversial and polemical critic of the most diverse topics, such as education, transportation and health [12]. Due to disagreements with the Catholic Church, which also did not skimp on its critical approaches, he ended up leaving the priesthood in 1969 [11]. Most importantly, he wrote books and defended innovative and radical ideas in the field of education. In the health area, he used his restless and brilliant mind for a remarkable reflection, materialized in the publication, in 1974, of the work '*Medical Nemesis*' also known, in a 1975 reissue, as '*Limits to Medicine*', [1], where makes a forceful criticism, revealing original points of view at the time, to the phenomenon of "medicalization" that was beginning to become evident and that he qualified as "pernicious medicalization of health".

3. From medicalization to Iatrogenesis

The term "medicalization" (which has not yet been included in the main Brazilian dictionaries) can be considered a polysemic word, if not with different meanings, but certainly with different connotations. Some authors even associate the term with a positive attribute, as in the case of AIDS, when the entire health production chain mobilized, in an unusual way until then, to understand the etiology of the disease, learn to diagnose and develop treatments, first to avoid deaths and then to prolong life and to provide greater well-being to people affected by the referred disease [13].

In his approach, Illich made no concessions to the eventual positive aspect of what he called the "medicalization of life", which he called as unhealthy for producing a "morbid society".

Continuing in his critique on "medicalization", he found that epidemiologists were unable to prove, for example, that early intervention altered the survival rate of patients affected by breast cancer. Likewise, he questioned the treatments for lung cancer, whose medical interventions brought more expenses and more suffering, without changing the survival rate - constantly mentioning the studies and articles that supported his conclusions [1].

It was also worth using drug treatments as an example, stating that the evaluation of the advantages (benefits) and disadvantages (undesired effects) caused by the drugs could be null or even negative, an aspect that even today seems to remain unnoticed, if not neglected.

This preamble on "medicalization" was used by Illich in his book to make way towards the concept of iatrogenesis, formed by the Greek words iatros (doctor) and genesis (origin). He thus defined iatrogenic disease as one that characterizes all the clinical conditions of which physicians, drugs, laboratories or hospitals - any medical apparatus, anyways, are pathogenic agents.

4. Social Iatrogenesis

In the chapter he called Social Iatrogenesis, Illich dealt with issues that are still disturbing today and that are frequently addressed in the field of public health.

He affirmed, for example, that "the level of health did not improve even when medical expenses increased", and was supported by studies that showed that although the USA allocated a considerable percentage of its GDP in the health system (7.4%, in 1974), they were not able to obtain good indicators, because the life expectancy of adult men paradoxically declined in that country [1].

The percentage of GDP invested in health by the United States in health reached an incredible 17.1% in 2013 [14]. Although health expenditures in that country lead the world statistics by far, however, Americans, as Illich emphasized, are not able to obtain a counterpart in health indicators, as for example, the life expectancy at birth (79 years) where they appear in the 34th position [14].

It is worth mentioning, based on this evident American paradox,, a vernacular created by Illich, "counterproductivity" [15], which he defined as "the paradoxical effect of overproduction and overconsumption", to verify and exemplify that the global volume of vehicles, designed to allow greater speed in travel, ends up stopping circulation on the roads public; the global volume of education prevents children from expanding their curiosity, intellectual courage and sensitivity; and that the global volume of "medicalization" reduces the level of health (ILLICH, 1975, p. 70).

No less interesting, still to characterize the "medicalization" of society, it was the record that the author already made at that time about the wonder that technology caused in people, impelling them to believe that health increased as they had access to prostheses, drugs, hospitalizations and examinations for preventive controls.

A similar finding was recorded, more than twenty years later, by the American cardiologist Bernard Lown, who was discouraged after investing a lot of time in the collection of a detailed medical history, which gave him exactly the diagnosis, to see that the patient appears to be incredulous. But when he took him to an examination room, where he had an old-fashioned fluoroscope with an image intensifier, with an instrument panel similar to that of an airplane, he saw the patient impressed and saying with his buttons: "Ah, how nice it is to be in such a well-equipped medical office." Dr. Lown concludes, without hiding the nonconformity, that "the puerile faith in the magic of technology is one of the reasons why the public has been tolerating the dehumanization of medicine" [16].

In a recent publication, Atul Gawande, when dealing with aging and end-of-life care, also identifies the fetish that technology awakens in people, who are not encouraged to seek advice from a geriatrician, but who await with unquestionable expectation the invention of a device that doctors implant in them, for example, in the chest, hoping to reduce discomfort and prevent them from ending up, dependent on care, in a nursing home [17].

In general, it is common for people not to feel treated if the doctor does not request for an examination or does not prescribe a drug. On the contrary, they value the use of technologies, preferably the most up-to-date and sophisticated ones, without awareness of the iatrogenesis that tests and medications so often provoke.

"Medicalization" also reveals itself as a true outsourcing of care for one's own health, when people renounce the possibility of taking preventive care, eliminating bad habits, to surrender to the medical arsenals, the side effects of medicines and imaging tests, in addition to choosing hospitals as a safe place to obtain health, forgetting the risk of exposure to nosocomial infection, iatrogenesis of the most harmful.

Illich was radical and rebellious in renouncing "medicalization", so coherent and determined in his conviction, that he suffered for ten years from a brain tumor, the cause of his death, giving up the therapies available at the time, using only opiates to relieve the pain and accepting to live with a huge bulge on his right face that even startled his interlocutors [18].

5. Drug iatrogenesis and its consequences

Iatrogenesis caused by drugs is usually studied based on factors related to the prescription: whether it is foreign to the therapeutic relationship; if it is at odds with the clinical diagnosis; whether the doses or duration of treatment are inadequate; whether undesirable, harmful or unexpected effects occur; if there is morbidity or mortality and if interactions between drugs occur that are harmful to the patient [19]. In addition, iatrogenic episodes occur even when prescriptions follow clinical protocols and drug labels, for the simple reason that people do not react in the same way, even if they have the same diagnoses.

In addressing some causes of iatrogenesis caused by drugs, Illich highlighted some factors not directly linked to the doctor-patient relationship as described above, but to other external aspects, such as the role of the pharmaceutical industry, whether in spending on advertising and commercial promotion with doctors, but mainly in stimulating the overconsumption of medicines, which increases the potential for damage related to the intake of medicines.

These aspects are still a current phenomenon and have been echoed by several authors, who denounce even the manipulation of academic studies, the creation of diseases that no longer admit any healthy individual [20], treating as medical problems which are non-medical [13], inventing diseases to sell their drugs [21], even considering that "a healthy person is just an undiagnosed patient" [22].

The laboratories' obsession with increasing the consumption of medications seems to have no limit, as can be seen in the encouragement of prescription classified as off label, when manufacturers convince doctors to prescribe drugs for indications other than those approved regulatory agencies at the time of their registration. The pharmaceutical industry does this by preparing articles and paying researchers to put their names in these "studies", with the explicit aim of increasing sales, as Marcia Angell, a Harvard professor, reported in a hard-hitting publication [23].

In 'Medical Nemesis', Illich pointed out that 3 to 5% of all hospitalizations in the United States of America (USA) had as a main reason, bad drug reaction. And that, once hospitalized, 18 to 30% of patients experienced an adverse reaction caused by a drug substance, doubling the length of hospital stay (ILLICH, 1975, p. 25).

The consultation of more recent studies confirms the relevance of this relationship, as was verified in the assessment of patient admissions in the Department of Cardiology and Pulmonology, in a large hospital in the Netherlands [24]. The authors conclude, after evaluating 2,000 hospitalizations by pharmacists and epidemiologists, that 19% of hospital admissions were motivated by adverse drug reactions (using the World Health Organization definition for this type of occurrence) and this percentage may reach 29% if hospitalizations classified as possibly iatrogenic are also considered.

An observational study carried out at a University Hospital in Spain sought to estimate the prevalence of negative results associated with drugs as a cause of hospitalization, by means of a random choice carried out by lot, which resulted in the analysis of 163 patients [25]. In 16.6% of the studied cases (27 patients) admission to the hospital was caused mainly by an adverse reaction due to use of the drug, of which 88.9% were considered preventable. The study concluded that hospitalizations motivated by an adverse reaction to medications had a high prevalence and most would be preventable through pharmacotherapeutic follow-up.

Another cross-sectional study, also conducted in Spain, evaluated patients who were hospitalized from the emergency services of a hospital. We sought to assess the negative results associated with the use of drugs that motivated hospitalization, to know the drugs that appeared more frequently and to assess the economic impact of these occurrences [26]. The conclusion was that 19.4% of hospitalizations occurred as a direct consequence of negative clinical results associated with the use of drugs, 65% of which were considered preventable. In addition, it was observed that the antineoplastic and immunosuppressive therapy groups motivated 38% of these adverse reactions. It was also found that 20.4% of the patients needed to be treated in an intensive care unit. Finally, it was found that the expense incurred was 237,377 euros (estimated annualized cost of 15,568,952 euros).

In the case of illnesses caused by Adverse Drug Events (ADE), in a meta-analysis 39 studies were selected (out of a total of 153) that evaluated the incidence of severe or even fatal ADE in American hospitals [27]. The conclusion was that the incidence of serious (6.7%) and fatal events (0.32%) was considered expressively high. Although the authors of the study noted the caveat that the results should be viewed with caution, because of the heterogeneity between the studies and possible bias in the samples, they warn that these data suggest that the adverse reaction to drugs represents an important health problem public in the United States of America (USA).

In a review article on adverse events (AE) in medical and hospital care, it was noted that ADEs are the most frequently identified, in addition to being also the most underreported [28]. In another evaluation carried out in a teaching hospital, which sought to estimate the frequency of this occurrence, it was observed that 14.6% of the 240 hospitalizations evaluated were motivated by ADE [29].

In England, a prospective observational study conducted in two large general hospitals sought to assess the cause of hospitalization in 18,820 patients hospitalized over a six-month period, seeking to identify which of these admissions were due to ADE, in addition to other aspects related to them. The prevalence obtained was 6.5% (1,225 cases), with 80% of this total directly related to an adverse drug reaction. The study concludes that this is an important problem considering morbidity, mortality and extra costs attributed to the studied events [30].

In Brazil, an original study focused on hospital admissions related to intoxication and adverse effects of drugs in children under one year of age. The retrospective analysis of the Authorizations for Hospital Admissions (AHA) of the Unified Health System (SUS), from 2003 to 2005, identified that a total of 1,063 children under one year of age were hospitalized as a direct or indirect consequence of drug-related intoxications or adverse effects [31].

Elderly patients are more susceptible to this type of occurrence due to the overuse and concomitant use of various drugs, administration errors and changes in the organism that interfere with pharmacodynamics and pharmacokinetics [32]. Although more vulnerable, the occurrence of iatrogenic disease in the elderly has not been studied in the dimension that the problem represents, since the population considered elderly is characterized by having multiple chronic diseases, is usually treated by many doctors and ends up being more subject to hospitalization and medical or surgical procedures [33].

Studies that analyze the relationship between pharmacotherapy and hospitalization of the elderly population also confirm that the occurrence rates are significantly high and are largely preventable [34]. Many of these hospital admissions for elderly patients are attributed to known drugs and occur because of drug interactions, which can also be prevented [35].

In the analysis of emergency hospitalizations for ADE in older adults, it was also found that they resulted from commonly used drugs and relatively few occurred due to the use of drugs considered to be high risk or inappropriate, which allows us to infer that such occurrences would also be preventable [36].

There are numerous studies that list hospital admissions due ADE and invariably conclude that we are facing an important public health problem, which not only reduces the patient's quality of life but generates unnecessary expenses for hospitals [37] and, consequently, for the health system. Although the hospitalizations that are attributed to ADE vary in relation to the percentage, the findings are always significant when studying the causes of hospitalizations [38].

Adverse reactions to medications, even in cases of diagnosis, prescriptions and correct administration, can be explained by the trial-and-error methodology, which is still decisive in medical practice.

It should be emphasized that the search for the definition of the most appropriate drug and dosage makes use of experimenting with people's reactions, and while pursuing the patient's benefit, it often produces harmful effects. In the next topic, the potential contributions of knowledge of genomics to mitigate the harmful effects of iatrogenesis caused by drugs and their possible repercussions on people and health systems will be discussed.

6. Pharmacogenetics

The sequencing of the human genome has revolutionized biology in several fields of study. Until 2012, 67% of global investments in genome sequencing technologies were directed to pure research and 11% to field of health. The projection for 2017 pointed out that investments in health would channel 39% of resources, mainly due to the reduction in the cost of exams and the applicability in medical practice, diagnosis and treatment [7]. That is, the field of health is the one that increasingly uses the potential of next generation sequencing.

The influence of genetics on how people react differently to drugs has been observed for at least five decades. Recent knowledge brought by genomics has an invaluable support potential to medicine, for doctors, geneticists and for the pharmaceutical industry, in the use of personalized treatments [39].

In the case of drugs, therapeutic inefficacy or pharmacological toxicity has frequently been observed due to the presence of some metabolizing enzymes in drugs, in which drugs can interfere as inhibitors or inducers of these enzymes, an activity that varies between individuals and that can be determined by DNA analysis [40]. Genetic variability, therefore, can affect how a drug can be absorbed, activated, metabolized or excreted from the organism [41].

The reaction to the same drug varies from person to person depending on weight, age, gender, liver and kidney function, interactions between drugs, type of disease and genetic factors. The drug goes through two major processes in the organism, called pharmacokinetics and pharmacodynamics. Pharmacogenetics seeks to study how the drug passes through these processes, establishing the link between metabolism and individual differences in people's DNA [42].

This metabolization can occur in different ways. In addition to the normal metabolizers, which respond as expected to the dosage of the package insert leaflet, there are slow metabolizers, which, due to reduced enzyme activity, are at risk of accumulating toxic levels and are more exposed to adverse reactions. Ultra-rapid metabolizers tend to require higher doses and are subject to the inefficacy of pharmacological therapy [41]. In addition, there is the intermediate metabolizer, which can benefit from the dose of the package insert leaflet but which can also be subject to the inefficacy of drug therapy.

The inclusion of genetic tests in the routine of medical practice is one of the main objectives of the *Clinical Pharmacogenetis Implementation Consortium (CPIC)*, a non-profit entity created to disseminate knowledge and issue guidelines on the use of genomic findings in drug prescriptions [43], which brings together the *PharmaGKB and Pharmacogenomics Research Network* [44].

CPIC defines the terms pharmacogenetics and pharmacogenomics, which are sometimes used interchangeably by some authors. Pharmacogenetics is the study of the genetic influence on the response to the drug, normally considering one or only a few genes involved. Pharmacogenomics is the study of the variation of how genomics influences the response to the drug, considering the sequencing of the entire human genome[1].

Pharmacogenetics emerged as a diagnostic tool that uses genetic information to guide pharmacotherapy decisions, improving the clinical outcome, giving rise to personalized clinical decisions [45].

These terms also differ according to their origin. Pharmacogenetic expression was coined by Friedrich Vogel in 1959 [46]. The word pharmacogenomics appears logically after the Human Genome Project.

Pharmacogenetics associates variability to drug response to hereditary aspects after the identification of some pharmacogenes [47]. Pharmacogenomics is one of the first clinical applications of the post-genomic era and expands this dimension to even point to the development of personalized drugs [48].

The following are some examples of the applicability of the use of pharmacogenetics in drug treatments widely used in psychiatry, cardiology and oncology.

7. Pharmacogenetics in psychiatry

The main causes of individual variability in response to the same dose of a drug are: age, biological factors, immunological factors, interactions between drugs and genetic factors [49]. Pharmacogenetics studies the role of genetics in variability of drug response.

This response can vary from potentially lethal adverse reactions to the equally serious lack of therapeutic efficacy.

Genetic variability plays an important role in pharmacokinetics (absorption, distribution, metabolism and excretion) and in pharmacodynamics, that is, in the interaction of the drug with the target and in the relationship between its concentration and its effect [50].

Currently, many studies are published that relate drugs to individuals' genetic variants. In psychiatry, in the case of initial treatment for depression, about 30 to 40% of patients do not respond adequately to the prescribed medication, and it can take up to six weeks to characterize that it is not effective [51], exposing the patient to a long period therapy based on trial and error, with a high chance of adverse reactions.

The use of knowledge of the presence of variants in the genes involved in the metabolism of antidepressants such as CYP2D6 can provide the physician with an important subsidy in the choice of medications and in the definition of the dosages used in the treatment of depression [52].

---

[1] PGKB – PharmGKB – The Pharmacogenomics Knowledgebase, available at https://www.pharmgkb.org/page/overview

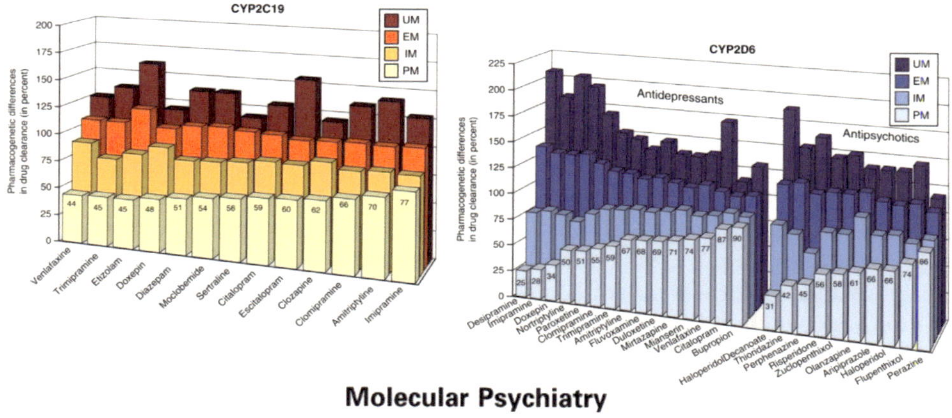

Figure 1.
Genetic variability of enzymes that metabolize drugs. Source: Molecular Psychiatry *(2013)* ***18****, 273–287; doi:10.1038/mp.2012.42.*

The genetic variability of the drug response, depending on the type of metabolizer, is very high, as shown in **Figure 1**, which shows the demonstration of the main marker genes (CYP2D6 and CYP2C19) for antidepressants and anxiolytics [53].

Considering the Extensive Metabolizer (MS) as one that obtains an adequate response with the dose of the package insert, the window of variability is very large in relation to the Ultra-Rapid Metabolizer (UM) and the Poor Metabolizer (PM), especially, as shown in **Figure 1** in the cases of the psychotherapeutic drugs, Escitalopram and Desipramine.

8. Pharmacogenetics in cardiology

Several important drugs used in the treatment of heart disease are already the subject of studies on pharmacogenetics, especially in anticoagulants, antihypertensive agents, antiarrhythmics and statins.

Warfarin is the most commonly used oral anticoagulant in the world and aims to prevent thromboembolism. Warfarin therapy is often associated with a high risk of increased bleeding, especially during the initial phase of treatment. The CYP2C9 gene is responsible for the metabolic degradation of the activity of this drug and the VKORC1 gene is responsible for the activation of vitamin K-dependent coagulation factors. When inhibiting VKORC1, Warfarin produces the anticoagulant effect [54].

Although the consequences of undue dosages are always serious, the dose of Warfarin is usually adjusted by the trial-and-error method, or by considering other clinical parameters obtained in conventional laboratory tests. The optimal dose of warfarin varies greatly between patients. If the dose is too strong, the risk of serious bleedings increases, and if it is too weak, the risk of stroke increases. It is estimated that two million Americans start treatment with warfarin annually [55].

A study that sought to describe the frequency and characteristics of ADEs, which led people to seek emergency care in the USA, concluded, among other findings, that the second drug that motivated the occurrence was warfarin, just behind the insulins [56].

Another study that evaluated the bleeding complications caused by the use of anticoagulants concluded that the drug has been used in an increasing proportion and that bleeding has been a predominant reaction, in addition to being an important cause of mortality [57].

From what we tried to describe, there is no doubt that we are dealing with a class of drugs (anticoagulants) of special relevance, which deserves all possible care in the prescription process, mainly due to the high potential for harm to patients and the cost it entails for the health system, as ADE almost always require hospital admissions.

In another case–control study in the USA, we sought to assess whether the genotyping test for patients starting warfarin treatment could reduce the incidence of hospitalizations due to bleeding or thromboembolism. Compared with the control group over a six-month period, one of the main conclusions was that genotyped patients had a 43% lower risk of hospitalization for bleeding or thromboembolism. The authors conclude that genotyping for the anticoagulant reduces the risk of hospitalization for hemorrhage or thromboembolism in patients who start outpatient treatment with warfarin, with great statistical and clinical significance. They further defend that doctors should seriously consider the use of pharmacogenetic tests for patients who are starting treatment with the referred drug [58].

It should also be noted that oral anticoagulants are among the most sensitive to drug interactions, especially when taken simultaneously with antidepressants [59]. In these cases, the influence of metabolization between drugs must be observed by clinicians and pharmacists, without obviously disregarding the adverse events arising from these interactions.

More recent studies seek to evaluate new algorithms that increase assertiveness in warfarin prescription. Such algorithms associate genetic variables with age, gender, body mass, vitamin K levels and thyroid function. At the current stage, studies should also be developed that also consider geographic areas and ethnic groups, in order to guarantee greater therapeutic efficacy, mitigate adverse reactions to the drug and reduce hospitalizations motivated by it [60].

In the case of statins, used in the control of cholesterol and in the prevention of cardiovascular diseases. Its use is widespread today, but the prescriptions ignore the effects of the presence of polymorphisms in the SLCO1B1 gene, in charge of synthesizing a family of proteins inside the cells for their metabolism and therapeutic action.

Several studies have been and are being carried out to verify how patients metabolize the different types of statins, some more or less indicated according to the phenotype of each individual, in order to avoid the side effects that in the case of statins are manifested mainly in myopathies that can worsen patients' living conditions.

Currently, at least 7 types of statins can be prescribed: atorvastatin, fluvastatin, lovastatin, pravastatin, pitavastatin, rosuvastatin and simvastatin. Although these different types share the same mechanism of action, they have differences in their chemical structures and pharmacokinetic profiles. Chemical structures end their solubility in water and influence the way they are absorbed, distributed, metabolized and excreted [61]. The patient can metabolize each of these different types of statins differently, an aspect that can be revealed by the pharmacogenetic test.

As an area responsible for the main cause of death in the world, drug therapy for Cardiovascular Diseases is the focus of attention in pharmacogenetic studies also for other drugs related to it. In addition to those already mentioned, there are plenty of studies relating genetic variants to the way we process antiplatelet drugs such as Clopidogrel, aspirins and antihypertensive drug [62].

9. Pharmacogenetics in oncology

Minimizing toxicity while maximizing efficacy is a common goal for the treatment of any condition, but its importance is even more evident in the case of oncology, due to the severe nature of the disorders and the aggressive toxicity caused by chemotherapeutic agents, in addition to the risk of relapse cancer or disease progression. The challenge of achieving an optimal therapeutic index is especially relevant for the elderly population, due to age-related changes in metabolism and the interaction with concomitant medications [63].

Over the past decade, advances in pharmacogenetics and pharmacogenomics have revealed the relationship between genetic variables and individual differences in drug responses. A large part of these advances has been made in the field of antineoplastic therapy.

Periodically, the American agency U. S. Food and Drug Administration (FDA) updates drug labels and edits table with related pharmacogenomic biomarkers. In 2016, 166 drugs (55 of them for cancer treatments) made up the table in which the FDA defines it as mandatory or in which it at least recommends the pharmacogenetic test, before the first prescription [64]. The variable reaction to drugs in the forms of unresponsiveness and adverse effect, and the motivation to use them better are the basis for one of the main objectives of the so-called personalized medicine, more recently disseminated as precision medicine.

10. Final considerations

Currently, iatrogenesis classified as adverse events, including those caused by drugs, are still an important public health problem, as has been demonstrated.

In response to the effects of these events, which are almost always harmful to people and those who offend the cost of assistance, pharmacogenetics, which emerged to improve the assertiveness of treatments to the point of being able to personalize them, may also contribute to minimize iatrogenesis, including the most serious ones requiring hospital admissions.

Although this goal is promising, there are still many challenges in implementing pharmacogenetic tests in clinical practice. First, concomitant factors such as diet, age and drug interactions affect pharmacokinetics and pharmacodynamics, increasing the complexity of assessing biomarkers in each patient. Second, the nature of the heterogeneity of clinical conditions presents a considerable therapeutic challenge. For example, in the case of cancer, treatment choices based on a biomarker present in a single biopsy sample may not be sufficient. Third, the definition of gene panels for each case is another area that needs to be developed, in order to facilitate the interpretation of clinicians [65].

The adoption of pharmacogenetic tests in routine clinical practice has been very scarce, particularly in Brazil. The main barriers to its implementation in the medical clinic are the lack of doctors' knowledge about the applicability in prescriptions, in addition to the provision of clear and accessible recommendations, based on proven evidence, as CPIC has been trying to do [66].

It is noteworthy that another difficulty of great relevance has been the lack of studies that demonstrate the positive cost-effectiveness of its application [67].

However, the continuous fall in the costs of sequencing allows us to project a not-too-distant future in which the realization of the exome (mapping the approximately 20,500 genes currently known), in early life, will allow a continuous revisit to the genetic results, which will be available and applicable in medical clinic for life [43], including the specificity of drug reaction.

The use of the findings of pharmacogenetics may not be a redeeming strategy in the solution of all drug iatrogeneses, reported more than forty years ago by Ivan Illich, because other factors, as mentioned here, interfere in the metabolism of drugs. But their adoption may significantly mitigate the deaths and suffering caused by them, in addition to replacing the practice of trial and error in prescriptions and dosimetry - a notable imperfection in medical practice and the health system.

Acknowledgements

Although the imperfections must all be credited to the author, I would like to put on record my utmost gratitude to Prof. Dr. Vera Lucia Luiza for the countless suggestions, tireless revisions and diligent guidance in the preparation of the article.

Author details

José Antonio Diniz de Oliveira[1,2]

1 Faculty of Public Health, University of São Paulo, Brazil

2 Escola Nacional de Saúde Pública Sergio Arouca, Oswaldo Cruz Foundation (ENSP/Fiocruz), Brazil

*Address all correspondence to: diniz@conectgene.com

References

[1] Illich I. NÊMESIS DA MEDICINA - A Expropriação da Saúde. 3a. Rio de Janeiro: Editora Nova Fronteira; 1975. 196 p.

[2] Alanazi MA, Tully MP, Lewis PJ. A systematic review of the prevalence and incidence of prescribing errors with high-risk medicines in hospitals. J Clin Pharm Ther. June 2016;41(3):239-245.

[3] Garfield S, Reynolds M, Dermont L, Franklin BD. Measuring the Severity of Prescribing Errors: A Systematic Review. Drug Saf. 2013;36:1151-1157.

[4] Lewis PJ, Dornan T, Taylor D, Tully MP, Wass V, Ashcroft DM. Prevalence, incidence and nature of prescribing errors in hospital inpatients: a systematic review. Drug Saf. 2009;32(5):379-389.

[5] Cunha GWB da. Iatrogenia caligráfica; a terrível doença da letra do médico. Hosp São Paulo. March 1986;10(37):17-18.

[6] Kalow W. Pharmacogenomics: historical perspective and current status. Pharmacogenomics Methods Protoc. 2005;3-15.

[7] Mohamed S, Syed BA. Commercial prospects for genomic sequencing technologies. Nat Rev Drug Discov. 2013;12(5):341-342.

[8] Henderson D, Barclay L. Strong Link Between Med Errors and Drug Class, Medical Unit [Internet]. Medscape. 2017 [mentioned on March 2, 2017]. Available at: http://www.medscape.com/viewarticle/875149

[9] Zaid G. Illich el removedor. Let Libr. 2011;(122):40-42.

[10] O'Mahony S. Medical Nemesis 40 years on: the enduring legacy of Ivan Illich. J R Coll Physicians Edinb. 2016;46(2):134-139.

[11] Hornedo B. Iván Illich. Hacia una sociedad convivencial [Internet]. Ivan Illich. 2004 [mentioned on November 24, 2015]. Available at: http://www.ivanillich.org.mx/vida.htm

[12] Gajardo M. Ivan Illich. PROSPECTS-UNESCO. 1993;23:711-711.

[13] Camargo Jr KR. Medicalização, farmacologização e imperialismo sanitário. Cad Saúde Pública. 2013;29(5):844-846.

[14] OMS. Organização Mundial de Saúde - Países [Internet]. OMS. 2014 [mentioned on March 21, 2016]. Available at: http://www.who.int/countries/en/

[15] Dupuy J-P. Ivan Illich ou la bonne nouvelle. Nous. 2002;2040:2050.

[16] Lown B. A arte perdida de curar. 2a. Editora Peirópolis; 2008. 352 p.

[17] Gawande A. Mortais. 1a. Editora Objetiva Ltda.; 2015. 259p.

[18] Kempf H. La mort d'Ivan Illich, penseur rebelle. Le Monde. May 12, 2002;13.

[19] Sougey EB, de Carvalho TFR. Iatrogenia dos medicamentos. Rev Bras Med Psicossomática. 1997;1(2):72-75.

[20] Machado LV, Ferreira RR. A indústria farmacêutica e a psicanálise diante da "epidemia da depressão": respostas possíveis. Psicologia em Estudo. 2014;19(1):135-144.

[21] Cassels A, Moynihan R. Pour vendre des médicaments, inventons des maladies. Le Monde diplomatique. May 2006;34 e 35.

[22] Orueta Sánchez R, Santos Rodríguez C, González Hidalgo E, Fagundo Becerra EM,

Alejandre Lázaro G, Carmona de la Morena J, et al. Medicalización de la vida (I). Rev Clínica Med Fam. 2011;4(2):150-161.

[23] Angell M, Barcellos W. A verdade sobre os laboratórios farmacêuticos. Rio de Janeiro: Record; 2007.

[24] Atiqi R, van Bommel E, CleophasTJ, ZwindermanAH. Prevalence of iatrogenic admissions to the Departments of Medicine/Cardiology/Pulmonology in a 1,250 bed general hospital. Int J Clin Pharmacol Ther. 07PY - 2010 de 2010;48(8):517-24.

[25] Santamaría-Pablos A, Redondo-Figuero C, Baena MI, Faus MJ, Tejido R, Acha O, et al. Resultados negativos asociados con medicamentos como causa de ingreso hospitalario. Farm Hosp. 2009;33(1):12-25.

[26] Pérez Menéndez-Conde C, Bermejo Vicedo T, Delgado Silveira E, Carretero Accame E. Resultados negativos asociados al uso de medicamentos que motivan ingreso hospitalario. Farm Hosp. 10PY - 2011 de 2011;35(5):236-43.

[27] Lazarou J, Pomeranz BH, Corey PN. Incidence of Adverse Drug Reactions in Hospitalized Patients. A Meta-analysis of Prospective Studies. J Am Med Assoc. April 15, 1998;279(15).

[28] Pedrosa TMG, Couto RC. Erros e eventos adversos na assistência médico hospitalar. Rev Médica Minas Gerais [Internet]. 2014 [mentioned February 15, 2016];24(2). Available at: http://www.gnresearch.org/doi/10.5935/2238-3182.20140054

[29] Cano FG. Eventos adversos a medicamentos no ambiente hospitalar [Internet]. [Rio de Janeiro]: Escola Nacional de Saúde Pública Sergio Arouca; 2011 [mentioned on November 11, 2015]. Available at: https://www.google.com.br/webhp?sourceid=chrome-instant&ion=1&espv=2&ie=UTF-8#q=eventos%20adversos%20a%20medicamentos%20no%20ambiente%20hospitalar

[30] Pirmohamed M, James S, Meakin S, Green C, Scott AK, Walley TJ, et al. Adverse drug reactions as cause of admission to hospital: prospective analysis of 18 820 patients. Bmj. 2004;329(7456):15-19.

[31] Lessa M de A, Bochner R. Análise das internações hospitalares de crianças menores de um ano relacionadas a intoxicações e efeitos adversos de medicamentos no Brasil. 2008 [mentioned on January 5, 2017]; Available at: http://www.arca.fiocruz.br/handle/icict/1320

[32] Paula TC de, Bochner R, Montilla DER. Clinical and epidemiological analysis of hospitalizations of elderly due to poisoning and adverse effects of medications, Brazil from 2004 to 2008. Rev Bras Epidemiol. December 2012;15(4):828-844.

[33] Permpongkosol S. Iatrogenic disease in the elderly: risk factors, consequences, and prevention. Clin Interv Aging. March 2011;77.

[34] Payot I. Problèmes reliés à la pharmacothérapie comme cause d'hospitalisation chez la personne âgée en perte d'autonomie [Internet]. [Genebra, Suíça]: Université de Genève; 2006 [mentioned on January 14, 2016]. Available at: https://doc.rero.ch/record/6430/files/these-PayotI.pdf

[35] Juurlink DNJ, Ma,dani MM, Kopp A, Laupacis A, Redelmeier DA. Drug-drug interactions among elderly patients hospitalizes for drug toxicity. J Am Med Assoc. April 2, 2003;289(13):1652-1658.

[36] Budnitz DS, Lovegrove MC, Shehab N, Richards CL. Emergency

hospitalizations for adverse drug events in older Americans. N Engl J Med. 2011;365(21):2002-2012.

[37] Varallo FR. Internações hospitalares por Reações Adversas a Medicamentos (RAM) em um hospital de ensino. 2010 [mentioned on February 4, 2016]; Available at: http://repositorio.unesp.br/handle/11449/96254

[38] Chaio S, Toibaro J, Valicenti P, Saidón P. Reacciones adversas medicamentosas y errores de prescripción: morbi-mortalidad. Med B Aires. 2013;73(2):111-118.

[39] Meyer UA. Pharmacogenetics - five decades of therapeutic lessons from genetic diversity. Nature Reviews Genetics. 2004;5:669-676.

[40] Lares-Asseff I, Trujillo-Jiménez F. La farmacogenética y su importancia en la clínica. Gac Med Mex. 2001;137(3):227-236.

[41] Brito M. A farmacogenética e a medicina personalizada. Saúde Tecnol. 2015;(14):5-10.

[42] Botelho JALM, Schpector JZ, Rodrigues N, Jr. EM. Avaliação da efetividade na distribuição de estatinas e antidepressivos no âmbito de um programa de distribuição de medicamentos de empresa de autogestão em saúde nas cidades de Campinas e Ribeirão Preto no Estado de São Paulo. [Programa de Pós-Graduação]. [São Carlos, SP]: Universidade Federal de São Carlos - UFSCAR; 2015.

[43] Relling MV, Evans WE. Pharmacogenomics in the clinic. Nature. October 14, 2015;526(7573):343-350.

[44] CPIC: Clinical Pharmacogenetics Implementation Consortium [Internet]. 2017 [mentioned on January 5, 2017]. Available at: https://www.pharmgkb.org/page/cpic

[45] Catalano M. The challenges of psychopharmacogenetics. Am J Hum Genet. 1999;65(3):606-610.

[46] Müller DJ, Rizhanovsky Z. From the Origins of Pharmacogenetics to First Applications in Psychiatry. Pharmacopsychiatry. July 2020;53(4):155-161.

[47] Campion DP, Dowell FJ. Translating Pharmacogenetics and Pharmacogenomics to the Clinic: Progress in Human and Veterinary Medicine. Front Vet Sci [Internet]. 2019 [mentioned on December 15, 2020];6. Available at: https://www.frontiersin.org/articles/10.3389/fvets.2019.00022/full

[48] Swen JJ, Huizinga TW, Gelderblom H, Vries EGE de, Assendelft WJJ, Kirchheiner J, et al. Translating Pharmacogenomics: Challenges on the Road to the Clinic. PLOS Med. August 14, 2007;4(8):e209.

[49] Rang HP, Dale MM. Rang and Dale's Pharmacology. Elsevier Brasil; 2007. 850 p.

[50] Weinshilboum RM, Wang L. Pharmacogenetics and pharmacogenomics: development, science, and translation. Annu Rev Genomics Hum Genet. 2006;7:223-245.

[51] Doris A, Ebmeier K, Shajahan P. Depressive Illness. The Lancet. 1999;(354):1369-1375.

[52] Lima IVM, Sougey EB, Vallada Filho HP. Farmacogenética do tratamento da depressão: busca de marcadores moleculares de boa resposta aos antidepressivos. Arch Clin Psychiatry São Paulo. 2004;31(1):40-43.

[53] Stingl JC, Brockmöller J, Viviani R. Genetic variability of drug-metabolizing enzymes: the dual impact on psychiatric therapy and regulation of brain function. Mol Psychiatry. March 2013;18(3):273-287.

[54] Pavani A, Naushad SM, Rupasree Y, Kumar TR, Malempati AR, Pinjala RK, et al. Optimization of warfarin dose by population-specific pharmacogenomic algorithm. Pharmacogenomics J. August 2012;12(4):306-311.

[55] McWilliam A, Lutter RW, Nardinelli C. Health care savings from personalizing medicine using genetic testing: the case of warfarin [Internet]. AEI-Brookings Joint Center for Regulatory Studies Washington, DC; 2006 [mentioned on February 27, 2016]. Available at: http://pgxlab.com/wp-content/uploads/2012/06/Health-Care-Savings-from-Personalizing-Medicine_AEI-Brookings.pdf

[56] Budnitz DS, Pollock DA, Weidenbach KN, Mendelsohn AB, Schroeder TJ, Annest JL. National surveillance of emergency department visits for outpatient adverse drug events. Jama. 2006;296(15):1858-1866.

[57] Wysowski DK, Nourjah P, Swartz L. Bleeding complications with warfarin use: a prevalent adverse effect resulting in regulatory action. Arch Intern Med. 2007;167(13):1414-1419.

[58] Epstein RS, Moyer TP, Aubert RE, O'Kane DJ, Xia F, Verbrugge RR, et al. Warfarin Genotyping Reduces Hospitalization Rates. J Am Coll Cardiol. June 2010;55(25):2804-2812.

[59] Teles JS, Fukuda EY, Feder D. Varfarina: perfil farmacológico e interações medicamentosas com antidepressivos. Einstein 16794508 [Internet]. 2012 [mentioned on January 5, 2017];10(1). Available at: http://search.ebscohost.com/login.aspx?direct=true&profile=ehost&scope=site&authtype=crawler&jrnl=16794508&AN=75332039&h=v%2B7aey3ySD9cv2T5Qr4V3xpQS9Iajqm5WroHX40Xxvwy3acDrIuzxoehJ1%2F%2BYXFXguIVGfVhe0NrkBzU7wMfMQ%3D%3D&crl=c

[60] Pavani A, Naushad SM, Kumar RM, Srinath M, Malempati AR, Kutala VK. Artificial neural network-based pharmacogenomic algorithm for warfarin dose optimization. Pharmacogenomics. January 2016;17(2):121-131.

[61] Gómez PG. SLCO1B1 gene variation and response to statin treatment. Trab Final Curso Grad. 2020;26.

[62] Zaiou M, El Amri H. Cardiovascular pharmacogenetics: a promise for genomically-guided therapy and personalized medicine. Clin Genet. March 01, 2017;91(3):355-370.

[63] Walko CM, McLeod HL. Personalizing Medicine in Geriatric Oncology. J Clin Oncol. August 20, 2014;32(24):2581-2586.

[64] FDA. Table of Pharmacogenomic Biomarkers in Drug Labeling [Internet]. EUA: U. S. Food and Drug Administration; 2016 [mentioned on February 18, 2016] p. 1-14. Available at: http://www.fda.gov/Drugs/ScienceResearch/ResearchAreas/Pharmacogenetics/ucm083378.htm

[65] Weng L, Zhang L, Peng Y, Huang RS. Pharmacogenetics and pharmacogenomics: a bridge to individualized cancer therapy. Pharmacogenomics. February 2013;14(3):315-324.

[66] E Caudle K, E Klein T, M Hoffman J, J Muller D, Whirl-Carrillo M, Gong L, et al. Incorporation of pharmacogenomics into routine clinical practice: the Clinical Pharmacogenetics Implementation Consortium (CPIC) guideline development process. Curr Drug Metab. 2014;15(2):209-217.

[67] Huang RS, Dolan ME. Approaches to the discovery of pharmacogenomic markers in oncology: 2000-2010-2020. Pharmacogenomics. April 2010;11(4):471-4.

Section 3

Impact of Pharmacogenetics on Different Diseases

Chapter 5

Pharmacogenetics of Direct Oral Anticoagulants

Natalia Shnayder, Marina Petrova, Elena Bochanova, Olga Zimnitskaya, Alina Savinova, Elena Pozhilenkova and Regina Nasyrova

Abstract

For more than 50 years, oral vitamin K antagonists were the choice of anticoagulant for the long-term treatment and prevention of arterial and venous thromboembolic events. In recent years, four direct oral anticoagulants (DOACs), dabigatran, rivaroxaban, apixaban and edoxaban have been compared with warfarin for thromboembolism prevention. These anticoagulants directly inhibit specific proteins within the coagulation cascade; in contrast, oral vitamin K antagonists inhibit the synthesis of vitamin K-dependent clotting factors. Dabigatran, a direct thrombin inhibitor, and rivaroxaban, apixaban and edoxaban, the factor Xa inhibitors, produce a more predictable, less labile anticoagulant effect. DOACs do not have limitations inherent vitamin K antagonists. DOACs have a predictable pharmacokinetic profile and are free of advers drugs reactions inherent in vitamin K antagonists. However, it is necessary to take into account the pharmacogenetic characteristics of the individual that can affect effectiveness and safety of use of DOACs. The results carried out to the present fundamental and clinical studies of DOACs studies demonstrate an undeniable the influence of genome changes on the pharmacokinetics and pharmacodynamics of DOACs. However, the studies need to be continued. There is a need to plan and conduct larger studies in various ethnic groups with the inclusion of sufficient associative genetic studies of the number of patients in each of the documented groups treatments with well-defined phenotypes.

Keywords: dabigatran etexilate, dabigatran, rivaroxaban, apixsaban, edoxaban, pharmacogenetics, effectiveness, safety, single nucleotide variant, CES1, ABCB1, ABCG2, CYP3A5, CYP2C9, CYP2J2, SLCO1B1, UGT1A9, UGT2B7, UGT2B15

1. Introduction

Thromboembolism (such as stroke and systemic embolism) is a serious complication of non-valvular atrial fibrillation (AF) [1]. Pulmonary embolism (PE) can cause death within first 14 days after a stroke in 25–50% of cases [2]. In absence of preventive measures, venous thromboembolic complications in lower limb arthroplasty (deep vein thrombosis and PE) reached 15–30% of cases before widespread use of anticoagulant therapy in clinical practice. However, with introduction of new anticoagulants in 2001, these indicators decreased to 1–2% [3], and in recent years-to 0.7–1.7% of [4]. Long-term use of anticoagulants is necessary for prevention of thromboembolic complications in patients with high risk of thromboembolism. For long time, vitamin K antagonists (warfarin, acenocumarol, phenindione) and indirect thrombin inhibitors (heparins) were used as drugs to prevent occurrence of thromboembolic complications [5, 6]. However, despite its effectiveness, coumarin therapy has some limitations. Drugs of this group are characterized by delayed therapeutic effect (after 36–72 hours from start of administration, with development of maximum effect on 5–7 days from start of use) [7]. Also, there is a need for regular therapeutic drug monitoring with the control of international normalized ratio (INR) indicator at safe level within 2–3, which entails additional economic burdens on health system [8]. A significant disadvantage of this group of drugs is irreversibility of drug in the event of an overdose [9]. The deviation of the INR from the permissible limits, both in lower and in higher direction, is prognostically unfavorable indicator. In first case, the therapeutic effect of anticoagulant therapy will not be achieved. In second case, the risk of hemorrhagic complications increases [10]. Balancing the effectiveness and safety of anticoagulant therapy is a difficult task in real clinical practice. Genetically determined features of individual's enzyme systems involved in drug metabolism make significant contribution to their effectiveness and safety [11]. An alternative to vitamin K antagonists were direct oral anticoagulants (DOACs), which do not have limitations inherent in warfarin [12]: dabigatran, rivaroxaban, apixaban, endoxaban. DOACs have a predictable pharmacokinetic profile and are free of disadvantages inherent in vitamin K antagonists. However, it is necessary to take into account the pharmacogenetic characteristics of the individual that can affect effectiveness and safety of use of DOACs.

2. Dagibatran

Dabigatran etexilate is first DOAC that has direct reversible inhibitory effect on thrombin [13, 14]. Thrombin is catalyst for conversion of factors V, VIII and XI in blood clotting cascade, and also catalyzes conversion of fibrinogen to fibrin and factor XIII to factor XIIIa, which contributes to stabilization of fibrin [15]. Also, thrombin activates GPCR receptors, which leads to conformational changes in platelets and promotes their aggregation. This leads to the release of even more clotting factors and the formation of more thrombin [16].

After entering the human body, dabigatran etexilate, being an inactive precursor (prodrug), quickly turns into an active metabolite – dabigatran. Dabigatran reversibly binds to the active center of the thrombin molecule, preventing thrombin-mediated activation of clotting factors. An important feature of dabigatran is that it can inactivate thrombin, even if it is in a bound state with fibrin [17]. The maximum concentration (Cmax) of dabigatran in plasma and, accordingly, anticoagulant action is observed as early as 0.5–2 hours after oral administration [18]. The half-life (T 1/2) of dabigatran with a single dose is 11 hours, but with regular intake it increases to 12–14 hours, which allows you to prescribe dabigatran etexilate 2 times a day [19]. Approximately one-third of the dabigatran circulating in blood binds to proteins. The drug is excreted unchanged from the body: 85% - with kidneys, 15% - with bile [20, 21].

It is important that dabigatran etexilate is not metabolized by cytochrome P450 isoenzymes of liver and does not change their activity. The CES1 and CES2 enzymes are human liver carboxylesterases that hydrolyze various xenobiotics and endogenous substrates using ester or amide bonds. Conversion of dabigatran etexylate to dabigatran depends more on activity of CES1 than on activity of CES2 [22–24].

Glycoprotein P (P-gp) is an ATP-dependent transporter that is involved in transfer of substrate molecules across membranes of expressing cells and components (regardless of concentration gradient) [25, 26]. P-gp is widely present in human body tissues and plays leading role in pharmacokinetics of dabigatran etexilate, which is a substrate for P-gp [13]. It is necessary to take into account drug interaction when prescribing dabigatran etexilate with P-gp inhibitors (verapamil, amiodarone, carvedilol, quinidine, spironolactone, nicardipine, propafenone, atorvastatin, clarithromycin, erythromycin, fluoroquinolones, ketoconazole, intraconazole, cyclosporine, fluoxetine, paroxetine, pentazocine, ritonavir, lopinavir, grapefruit juice, and others), as this leads to decrease in its effectiveness, increased absorption of these drugs, inhibition of their excretion, and increased penetration through barriers. This leads to an increase in the concentration of P-gp substrate drugs in the blood and tissues and increases the risk of adverse drug reactions (ADRs). Bernier et al. revealed development of bleeding in 30.4% of patients taking P-gp inhibitors together with dabigatran [27]. On contrary, drugs that are inducers of P-gp (rifampicin, morphine, dexamethasone, retinoids, barbiturates, nicotine, diphenin, isoniazid, carbamazepine, caffeine, diazepam, diphenhydramine, tricyclic antidepressants, phenytoin, ethanol), when used with dabigatran, by increasing activity of P-gp, lead to inhibition of dabigatran absorption, increase its elimination and inhibition of penetration through barriers. This leads to decrease in concentration of P-gp substrate drug and a decrease in its effectiveness. It is also important to take into account that simultaneous use of substrates and P-gp inhibitors increases the risk of developing congenital anomalies in fetus [28].

In addition to CES1 and ABCB1, which affect biotransformation of dabigatran etexylate and the effectiveness of active dabigatran, glucuronidation enzymes UGT2B15, UGT1A9, and UGT2B7 also participate in its metabolism (elimination). Their activity reflects safety of using dabigatran [29]. The main and most interesting enzyme involved in elimination of dabigatran is UGT2B15. When prescribing dabigatran etexilate, it is important to consider drug interactions with drugs that are metabolized by UGT2B15. By interacting competitively with enzyme, they can slow down metabolism of dabigatran (for example, acetaminophen, loratadine, lorazepam, oxazepam, morphine, valproic acid) [30, 31], and its concentration will increase, increasing the risk of ADRs.

To date, the *CES1* and *ABCB1* genes have been shown to have an important effect on metabolism of dabigatran etexilate, and single-nucleotide variants (ONVs) in these two loci probably play key role. There are many studies conducted worldwide to find out whether search for ONVs in *CES1* and *ABCB1* genes can explain some of inter-individual variability in the concentrations of the active metabolite dabigatran in the blood of humans, and *UGT2B15* gene may be potential candidate gene for safety studies of dabigatran. Paré et al. investigated the ONV of *CES1* gene to assess inter-individual profile of efficacy and safety of dabigatran as part of RE-LY (Randomized Evaluation of Long Term Anticoagulant Therapy study) [32]. Carriage of minor allele G (rs2244613) of *CES1* gene occurred in 32.8% of patients and was associated with minimal concentrations of dabigatran in the blood and, consequently, with a lower risk of bleeding ($p < 9 \times 10^{-8}$) [32]. Dimatteo et al. [33] found association of rs8192935 of *CES1* gene with a lower concentration of dabigatran in blood plasma ($p = 0.023$). Carriers of allele T showed significantly lower concentrations of dabigatran in blood plasma than carriers of homozygous CC genotype, which reduces the risk of hemorrhagic complications. Overall, the average plasma concentration of dabigatran was higher in patients with the CC genotype (86.3 ng/DL) than in patients with the allele T (62.1 ng/DL). At the same time, there was no significant effect of rs4148738 of *ABCB1* gene on concentration of dabigatran in blood [33].

Gouin-Thibault et al. [26] evaluated effect of clarithromycin on pharmacokinetics of dabigatran in 60 healthy male volunteers selected for *ABCB1* genotype (20 homozygous carriers of ONVs, 20 heterozygous and 20 homozygous carriers of the wild-type allele for haplotype 2677–3435). The results of the study AUC (Area Under the Curve – area under the curve) was 77% for dabigatran. The *ABCB1* genotype did not significantly affect pharmacokinetics of dabigatran: AUC ratio in carriers of studied ONVs and wild-type allele carriers was 1.27 (95% confidence interval (CI) 0.84–1.92), but clarithromycin administration led to twofold increase in AUC for dabigatran, regardless of *ABCB1* genotype: and was 2.0 (95% CI 1.15–3.60) [29].

The aim of the study is Shi et al. [24] studied effect of the ONVs of *CES1* gene and gender of patients on effectiveness of dabigatran using several in vitro approaches. Thus, 104 biopsy samples obtained from liver of patients of various racial backgrounds were examined for carriers of three ONVs: rs2244613, rs8192935, and rs71647871 or G428A, also referred to as G143E, which is variant of *CES1* with reduced enzymatic activity. The study showed that G143E is ONV with reduced metabolism for dabigatran. The activity of CES1 enzyme was significantly higher in female liver samples than in male liver samples. The data obtained by the authors indicate that the studied ONVs of *CES1* and the gender of patients are important risk factors contributing to variability of the pharmacokinetics of dabigatran etexilate in humans. A personalized approach to treatment with dabigatran etexilate should be based on identifying patient-specific genetic changes in the *CES1*. This approach can potentially improve the effectiveness and safety of pharmacotherapy with this drug [24].

The activity of glucuronidation enzymes depends on the ONVs of their encoding genes. To date, we have not found any works that would present studies of association of carrier of the UGT family genes on metabolism of dabigatran in humans. However, we can assume that this may change its concentration in blood plasma of patients. This hypothesis is based on previous studies of associations of ONVs carrier of *UGT2B15* gene on concentration of drugs that are metabolized in a similar way to dabigatran. He et al. [34] found that carriage of allele A (rs1902023) of the *UGT2B15* gene is associated with decrease in oxazepam clearance. In other words, in patients with this allele, glucuronidation of xenobiotics is slower, and concentration of drugs in blood plasma increases, thereby increasing the risk of developing ADRs [34]. A similar change in glucuronidation of drugs in carriers of this ONVs is shown for other drugs that are metabolized in similar way (lorazepam [31], acetominophen [35], tamoxifen [36], valproic acid [37]). In study of pharmacokinetics of cypoglitazarus Stringer et al. [38] showed that patients homozygous for UGT2B15*2 (rs1902023 G > T) had significantly higher concentrations of this drug in blood compared to patients carrying UGT2B15*1 genotypes/*2 or UGT2B15*1/*1 [38]. Thus, carrier is rs1902023 (UGT2B15*2) of *UGT2B15* gene is associated with delayed glucuronidation and is important predictor of interindividual variability in drug clearance. Therefore, this effect can have significant effect on metabolism of dabigatran as substrate of UGT2B15.

3. Rivaroxaban

Rivaroxaban is the first direct factor Xa inhibitor. Pharmacokinetics of rivaroxaban does not have disadvantages of vitamin K antagonists. However, pharmacokinetics and pharmacogenetics of rivaroxaban are variable. This can affect both effectiveness and safety of anticoagulant therapy.

Rivaroxaban inhibits platelet activation and fibrin clot formation by direct, selective and reversible inhibition of factor Xa in both intrinsic and extrinsic coagulation pathways. Factor Xa, as part of prothrombinase complex, also composed of factor Va, calcium ions, factor II, and phospholipids, catalyzes the conversion of prothrombin to thrombin. Thrombin activates platelets and catalyzes the conversion of fibrinogen to fibrin. Thus, factor Xa is a coagulation factor that acts at point of convergence of internal and external pathways in blood coagulation system. It catalyzes the breakdown of prothrombin and is therefore critical for thrombin generation. It is important to note that rivaroxaban inhibits free prothrombinase- and clot-associated factor Xa without directly affecting platelet aggregation [39]. This distinguishes rivaroxaban from indirect inhibitors of factor Xa, which does not inhibit factor Xa associated with prothrombinase complex [40].

When taken orally, rivaroxaban reaches its maximum plasma concentration after 2–4 hours. The absolute bioavailability of rivaroxaban for dosage of 10 mg is relatively high (80–100%) and does not depend on food intake [41, 42]. Under fasting conditions, oral bioavailability of rivaroxaban at dosage of 20 mg decreases to 66%. When using drugs at a dosage of 20 mg with food, the AUC increases to 39%. This indicates an almost absolute absorption and, at same time, a high oral bioavailability of rivaroxaban. The connection with plasma proteins reaches 92–95%. Because of this high plasma protein binding, rivaroxaban is not removed during dialysis [43].

Rivaroxaban is eliminated from body in various ways, of which three are main ones. Approximately 36% of dose is excreted unchanged by kidneys through active transporter-mediated secretion by P-glycoprotein (Pgp) and BCRP (ABCG2). In addition, 14% of dose is eliminated by hydrolysis of amide bonds and 32% of dose is eliminated via oxidative metabolic pathways. Liver isoenzymes CYP3A4 and CYP3A5 are responsible for metabolism about 18%, and CYP2J2 - about 14% of the dose [44, 45]. Level of rivaroxaban when administered concomitantly with midazolam (a CYP3A4 substrate) is reduced by an average of 11% compared with rivaroxaban alone. The following drugs moderately alter the level of rivaroxaban: erythromycin (a moderate inhibitor of CYP3A4/P-gp; an increase of 34%); clarithromycin (potent CYP3A4/mild P-gp inhibitor; 54% increase); fluconazole (moderate CYP3A4, a possible inhibitor of BCRP (ABCG2); an increase of 42%). A significant increase in blood levels and strength of action of rivaroxaban has been demonstrated when used simultaneously with drugs that are potent inhibitors of the CYP3A4 enzyme and P-gp/BCRP transporter proteins (ABCG2) and potential inhibitors of CYP2J2 enzyme, for example: use of ketoconazole 400 mg once a day leads to an increase in level of rivaroxaban by 158% (95% CI: 136% - 182%); the use of ritonavir increases level of rivaroxaban by 153% (95% CI: 134% - 174%) [46].

The expression of rivaroxaban transporter proteins may be influenced by SNVs of *ABCB1* gene, but information on their clinical significance is inconsistent. The systematic review and meta-analysis by Xie et al. [47] showed that Cmax was lower in carriers of *ABCB1* rs1045642 CC than carriers of TT, and carriers of rs2032582 GG than carriers of A/T allele, and AUC0-∞ was lower in rs1045642 CC carriers than in TT carriers [47]. In the study by Gouin-Thibault et al. [26] found that *ABCB1* polymorphisms is not significant determinant of individual variability in pharmacokinetics of rivaroxaban, and combined use of P-gp/CYP3A4 inhibitor clarithromycin with rivaroxaban may require caution in patients at risk of overdose, as it leads to two-fold increase in AUC genotype *ABCB1* [26].

In the study by Sychev et al. found no significant differences in peak steady-state concentration of rivaroxaban between mutant haplotypes and wild haplotypes of *ABCB1* gene [48]. The similar result was posted by Sennesael et al. [49]: ONVs 1236 C > T, −2677 G > T-3435, C > T and 1199 G > A of *ABCB1* gene did not significantly affect the intracellular accumulation of rivaroxaban compared to wild-type protein. These results suggest that *ABCB1* SNVs studied in present study are unlikely to contribute to individual variability in plasma rivaroxaban concentrations [49]. At same time, it was found that use of strong inhibitors and inducers of P-gp should be avoided in patients taking rivaroxaban [26, 50].

Promising direction is study of BCRP protein, encoded by *ABCG2* gene, which, like P-gp, provides absorption and excretion of rivaroxaban from intestinal lumen and renal tubules. The *ABCG2* gene is increasingly recognized as an important mediator of drug transport in the intestine and renal tubules [51], and its SNVs affect decrease in BCRP substrate transport in case of co-administration of rivaroxaban and other drugs [52]. Most studied SNVs in this gene, Q141K (rs2231142), is associated with decrease in ABCG2 activity and, consequently, with a decrease in activity of its drug substrates transport [53]. This SNVs has not yet been studied in context of pharmacogenetics of rivaroxaban; however, in an experimental mouse model, absence of P-gp (*ABCB1*) and BCRP (*ABCG2*) was associated with significantly reduced drug clearance [54].

Metabolism of rivaroxaban in liver is carried out by cytochrome P450 isoenzymes 3A4 (*CYP3A4*) and 2 J2 (*CYP2J2*), as well as by mechanisms independent of CYP [46]. To date, more than 50 SNVs of *CYP3A4* gene have been discovered, associated with different levels of activity of CYP3A4 isoenzyme. Associations between *CYP3A4* SNVs carriage and changes in pharmacological response have been described for atorvastatin, simvastatin, sacrolimus, and fentanyl [55]. Information on the change in pharmacological response of rivaroxaban in literature available to us was not found. At same time, it was found that use of strong inhibitors and inducers of CYP3A4 and P-gp should be avoided in patients taking rivaroxaban [50]. For example, "old" antiepileptic drugs (AEDs) that act on cytochrome P450 isozymes, and especially on CYP3A4, such as phenobarbital, phenytoin, and carbamazepine, are more likely to significantly reduce the anticoagulant effect of DOACs (especially rivaroxaban, apixaban, and edoxaban). New AEDs that do not significantly affect CYP or P-gp, such as lamotrigine or pregabalin, are unlikely to affect the effectiveness of DOACs. Zonisamide and lacosamide, which do not significantly interfere with in vitro CYP activity, may have a safe profile. However, their effect on P-gp has not yet been studied. Levetiracetam only has a potential effect on P-gp activity, so it may also be safe [56].

The study of effect of a potent P-gp inhibitor cyclosporin and its combination with a moderate CYP3A inhibitor fluconazole on pharmacokinetics of rivaroxaban and CYP3A activity (compared with baseline) showed that cyclosporine increased average exposure of rivaroxaban by 47%, maximum concentration of CYP3A4 and decreased by 34%, and cyclosporine in combination with fluconazole increased the average exposure of rivaroxaban by 86% and maximum concentration by 115%. This effect was significantly stronger than that observed in control group that received rivaroxaban with fluconazole alone [57].

The high clinical significance of interaction of rivaroxaban with other drugs is shown in a systematic review and meta-analysis of studies in which patients with atrial fibrillation were randomized to groups taking DOACs or warfarin, stratified by number of concomitant drugs [58]. Polypharmacy was significantly associated with poor outcomes and reduced the benefit in terms of risk of major bleeding in patients receiving rivaroxaban, especially in presence of drugs that modulate P-gp/CYP3A4.

Also, about 10 different SNVs for *CYP2J* gene are known, but their clinical role was mainly studied in the context of coronary heart disease (CAD) and arterial hypertension, since isoenzyme CYP2J encoded by this gene plays a role in the metabolism of arachidonic acid [59].

4. Apixaban

Apixaban is a potent direct oral reversible and highly selective factor Xa inhibitor that does not require antithrombin III for antithrombotic activity [60, 61]. Apixaban inhibits both free and clot-associated factor Xa and prothrombinase activity, which inhibits clot growth [62]. By inhibiting factor Xa, apixaban reduces formation of thrombin and development of blood clots. It has no direct effect on platelet aggregation, but indirectly inhibits thrombin-induced platelet aggregation [63].

Absorption of apixaban occurs mainly in small intestine and gradually decreases as it passes through it [64]. For oral doses up to 10 mg, absolute bioavailability of apixaban is about 50% due to incomplete absorption [65, 66] and first passage through liver [67, 68]. Apixaban Cmax in plasma is reached 3–4 hours after oral administration [69, 70]. Binding of apixaban to blood plasma proteins, mainly albumin, is about 87% [71]. After oral administration, unchanged apixaban is main drug component in human blood plasma without presence of active circulating metabolites [66]. Excretion of apixaban involves several pathways, including metabolism in liver, as well as excretion by unchanged parent compound in bile and kidneys, and direct intestinal excretion [72].

Metabolic pathways of apixaban include O-demethylation, hydroxylation, and sulfation of hydroxylated O-demethylapixaban [66]. At same time, metabolism mainly occurs through isoenzymes CYP3A4 /5 of liver cytochrome P450, with an insignificant participation of isoenzymes CYP1A2, CYP2C8, CYP2C9, CYP2C19 and CYP2J2 [67].

The role of non-functional allele G (rs776746) of *CYP3A5* gene has been most studied. At same time, in heterozygous carriers (genotype AG), metabolism of apixaban is moderately reduced due to carriage of one non-functional allele G, and in heterozygous carriers (CYP3A5 * 3, genotype GG) CYP3A5 isoenzyme is not expressed. This is a risk factor for development of ADRs (in particular, bleeding) when taking apixaban [73]. Ueshima et al. found that patients with AF and a homozygous TT genotype (rs77674) of *CYP3A5* gene may have decreased blood apixaban concentrations compared to patients with CC and CT genotypes. Therefore, carriage of allele T may be associated with an increased clearance of apixaban [73]. However, this study was conducted on patients from Asian population, which does not allow extrapolation of the results to other racial and ethnic groups.

The highest risk of developing apixaban-induced ADRs due to a slowdown in the metabolism of drug in liver, especially when combined with drugs-inhibitors of CYP3A5 isoenzyme, in homozygous carriers of non-functional alleles CYP3A5*2 (rs28365083), CYP3A5*3 (rs776746), CYP3A5*6 (rs10264272), CYP3A5*7 (rs41303343), CYP3A5*8 (rs55817950), CYP3A5*9 (rs28383479), CYP3A5*10 или CYP3A5*3 K (rs41279854), CYP3A5*11 (rs72552791), CYP3A5*3D (rs56244447), CYP3A5*3F (rs28365085), CYP3A5_3705C > T(H30Y) (rs28383468), CYP3A5_7298C > A(S100Y) (rs41279857). Among them, the most common is non-functional allele CYP3A5*3 (rs776746). In terms of phenotypes, individuals are "expressors" of CYP3A5 if they carry at least one CYP3A5*1 allele, and "non-expressors" if not. It should be noted that frequency of carriage of SNVs of CYP3A5 gene varies significantly depending on ethnicity of patients. For example, most Europeans are not expressors, while many people of African descent are CYP3A5 expressors [63, 74]. Higher concentrations of active component of drugs, metabolized with participation of isoenzyme CYP3A5, in blood plasma are higher in non-expressors of CYP3A5 compared with expressors [75]. In patients belonging to group of non-expressing CYP3A5 (homozygous carriers of the above non-functional alleles), apixaban dosing should be cautious and requires monitoring of ADRs. Co-administration of apixaban with other drugs metabolized with participation of CYP3A5 isoenzyme should be avoided in non-expressors,

The study SNVs of CYP3A5 gene was conducted among 200 postmenopausal women who had an episode of venous thromboembolism and more than 500 comparable control groups. It is known that oral estrogen intake increases the risk of venous thromboembolism in all women (odds ratio (OR) - 4.5; CI: 2.6–7). Compared with women who did not receive oral estrogens, the OR for venous thromboembolism in users of oral estrogens was 3.8 (CI: 2.1–6.7) among women who did not have the common (wild) CYP3A5 * 1 allele encoding a highly functional isoenzyme CYP3A5, and 30.0 (CI: 4.4–202.9) among patients with this allele (interaction test p = 0.04) [76]. This is important to consider when prescribing apixaban to postmenopausal women.

Carriage of low-functional alleles CYP1A2*1C (rs2069514), CYP1A2*1K_-729C > T (rs12720461), CYP1A2*1K_-739 T > G (rs2069526), CYP1A2*3 (rs56276452), CYP1A2*4A (rs56276455), CYP1A*4A (rs28399424) of *CYP1A2* gene leads to decrease in activity of CYP1A2 isoenzyme. This may be of clinical significance in long-term therapy with apixaban in homozygous carriers of low- or non-functional alleles of *CYP3A5* gene, due to the cumulative risk and disruption of auxiliary pathway of apixaban metabolism in the liver with the participation of the isoenzyme CYP1A2. This reduces metabolism of drug and increases the risk of ADRs. In addition, in carriers of CYP1A2*1C (rs2069514), concomitant use of apixaban with inhibitors of the isoenzyme CYP1A2 may slow down the breakdown of caffeine, which can lead to overstimulation by caffeine. On contrary, carriage of highly functional allele CYP1A2*1F (rs762551) can lead to an acceleration of apixaban metabolism. Smoking is a well-known CYP1A2 activator (especially in CYP1A2*1F carriers). This leads to a more rapid degradation of drugs metabolized with the participation of CYP1A2 isoenzyme, and possibility of insufficient concentration of drugs in body to obtain significant therapeutic benefits [77].

Carriers of SNVs of *CYP2C9* gene can metabolize drugs in different ways. From a clinical point of view, it is important of carriage of the following SNVs: rs1057910 (two variants that encode the "wild-type" CYP2C9*1 allele and the non-functional CYP2C9*3 allele), as well as rs1799853, rs9332131, rs72558190, rs72558 (non-functional variants CYP2C9*2, CYP2C9*6, CYP2C9*15, CYP2C9*25 respectively). In particular, the carriage of non-functional alleles CYP2C9*2 and CYP2C9*3 should be taken into account when co-administration of apixaban and clopidogrel, which inhibits the CYP2C9 isoenzyme in sufficiently high doses. This may affect the metabolism of drugs that are metabolized with the participation of the isoenzyme CYP2C9, and patients who are homozygous carriers of non-functional alleles of *CYP2C9* (slow metabolizers) are likely to be at greater risk of ADRs (in particular, the risk of bleeding) when taking clopidogrel and apixaban [78].

Some of major metabolic pathways of apixaban include o-demethylation, hydroxylation, and sulfation, with o-demethylapixaban sulfate being main metabolite [66]. Potentially important pharmacogenomic metabolic pathway is via sulfotransferases (SULT) SULT1A1 and SULT1A2, which are responsible for sulfation of o-demethyl-apixaban to o-demethyl-apixaban sulfate [79, 80]. SULT1A1 enzyme is more efficient than SULT1A2 in sulfation of o-demethyl-apixaban [81]. O-demethyl-apixaban is the most well-known metabolite and accounts for 25% of the estimated active apixaban [66]. It is important to know that o-demethyl-apixaban sulfate does not have any inhibitory activity against factor Xa, which may contribute to anticoagulant efficacy of apixaban [81]. Three important SNVs of *SULT1A1* gene have been described: SULT1A1*1 (wild type), SULT1A1*2 (rs9282861), and SULT1A1*3 (rs1801030) [80]. Vmax of all three allelic variants of *SULT1A1* gene (SULT1A1*1 > SULT1A1*3 > SULT1A1*2) varies, and this explains the differences in sulfation of active apixaban. The SULT1A*3 variant has a moderate potential to influence anticoagulant effect of apixaban, whereas SULT1A*2 has low potential to influence apixaban metabolism [82]. These different alloenzymes have different enzymatic efficiencies and can lead to different concentrations of metabolites and variations in anticoagulant efficacy of apixaban [83]. However, the effect of common genetic variants of *SULT1A1* gene on apixaban metabolism in patients has not yet been formally studied [78].

5. Edoxaban

Edoxaban is a selective, direct and reversible inhibitor of activated blood coagulation factor X (F Xa), a serine protease responsible for thrombin formation. Edoxaban is used to prevent stroke in nonvalvular AF, treat deep vein thrombosis and PE [84–86].

It binds to both free FXa and free FXa in prothrombinase complex, thus causing a dose-dependent decrease in thrombin formation [87].

Edoxaban is characterized by linear, predictable pharmacokinetic profile [88]. After oral administration, edoxaban reaches peak plasma concentrations (C max) within 1–2 hours [89]. The half-life (T1/2) of edoxaban is approximately 10–14 hours [88]. Edoxaban is absorbed mainly in upper gastrointestinal tract, approximately 13% is absorbed in large intestine [90].

In an in vitro study, five phase 1 metabolites of edoxaban were found in human liver microsomes: M-1, M-4, M-5, M-6 and a hydroxylated metabolite at the N-dimethylcarbamoyl group of edoxaban (hydroxymethylenedoxaban) (M-7) [91]. Formation of a metabolite M-4, unique for humans, is catalyzed by CES1, which is present in human liver microsomes and in the cytosol. Cytochrome P450 (CYP) 3A4 isoenzyme mediates formation of M-5 and hydroxymethylenedoxaban in presence of nicotinamide adenine dinucleotide phosphate (NADPH). It is assumed that M-8, minor metabolite, arises spontaneously (non-enzymatically) via an intermediary, hydroxymethylenedoxaban, which is formed via CYP3A4/5 [92].

Second phase of edoxaban metabolism is mediated by glucuronidation to form N-glucuronide metabolite (M-3). This metabolite has not been quantified. Three metabolites (M-4, M-6 and M-8) have anticoagulant activity with half-maximum inhibitory concentration (IC50) values for anti-FXa 1.8 nM (M-4), 6.9 nM (M-6) and 2.7 nM (M-8). The IC 50 value of edoxaban for anti-FXa is 3 nM [93]. However, due to its low content and high protein binding (80%), it is expected that most abundant metabolite M-4 will not make a significant contribution to overall pharmacological activity of edoxaban in patients with at least a moderate decline in renal function [94]. Other metabolites are present in even smaller amounts and (in the absence of liver cytochrome P450 inducers) do not significantly contribute to total anticoagulant activity of drugs. None of metabolic pathways alone contributes more than 10% to total clearance of edoxoban [92].

Edoxaban is a substrate for P-gp and is not a substrate for other transporters such as anion transport polypeptide (OATPs), 1B1, or organic cation transporters (OATs) 2 [95].

Edoxaban is mainly excreted unchanged in urine and through the secretion of biliary tract with feces [92]. Renal clearance of unchanged drugs is approximately 50% of total clearance, and remaining 50% of non-renal clearance occurs due to metabolism and secretion of the biliary tract. As previously described, edoxaban is metabolized by the enzymes CES1 (<10%), CYP3A4 (<10%) and by glucuronidation; but metabolism is a minor route of elimination of edoxaban in patients with normal renal function. Therefore, inhibitors or inducers of these enzymes are unlikely to have clinically significant interactions with edoxaban. However, drug interaction studies have been performed to investigate the effect of CYP3A4 inhibitors on the pharmacokinetics of edoxaban. In addition, the effects of other drugs that could be administered concurrently with edoxaban were evaluated. Since edoxaban is a substrate of the P-gp efflux transporter, several studies have been carried out on interaction of drugs with inhibitors, substrates and inducers of P-gp. The effect of co-administration of P-gp inhibitors was an increase in effect of edoxaban (maximum observed drug concentration in plasma C max and area under the curve of concentration versus time AUC), but the increase was less than 2 times. P-gp inhibitors and potent CYP3A4 / 5 inhibitors (eg, ketoconazole, erythromycin) do not result in greater increases in exposure compared to mild P-gp inhibitors (eg verapamil) or mild inhibitors (eg cyclosporine) CYP3A4 / 5. This confirms that the metabolism of CYP3A4/5 is not the main route of elimination of edoxaban [96, 97].

Co-administration of ketoconazole (P-gp inhibitor; potent CYP3A4 inhibitor) increased the single dose peak and overall exposure to edoxaban by 89% and 87%, respectively [98]. However, co-administration of oral quinidine (P-gp and OCT2 transporter inhibitor; potent CYP2D6 inhibitor) increased the single dose peak and 24-hour exposure of oral edoxaban by 85% and 77%, respectively [99].

Co-administration of sustained-release verapamil (P-gp inhibitor (main effect); moderate CYP3A4 inhibitor) increased the peak and 24-hour exposure of single doses of edoxaban by 53% [99].

Co-administration of erythromycin (P-gp inhibitor; moderate CYP3A4 inhibitor) increased the peak and total exposure of single doses of edoxaban by 68% and 85%, respectively [91]. Co-administration of cyclosporine (P-gp inhibitor, OATP1B1 and BCRP; weak inhibitor of CYP3A4) increased both the peak and total exposure of single doses of edoxaban by 74% and 73%, respectively [98]. Co-administration of dronedarone (a P-gp inhibitor) increased the peak and total exposure of single doses of edoxaban by 46% and 85%, respectively [99].

The administration of amiodarone (P-gp inhibitor; moderate CYP2C9 inhibitor, weak CYP2D6 inhibitor) to patients receiving edoxaban for 3 days of once daily administration increased the peak and total exposure of single doses of edoxaban by 66% and 40%, respectively [99]. This is important to remember because amiodarone has a long half-life, reaching an average of 58 days [100]. Rifampicin, inducer of P-gp (strong CYP3A4 inducer; moderate inducer of CYP2B6, 2C8, 2C9, 2C19; inhibitor of P-gp, OATP1B1, OATP1B3) after 7 days of dosing reduced the total exposure to edoxaban by about 34%, without affecting its peak exposure [101]. Co-administration of digoxin (P-gp substrate) increased the C max of edoxaban by 16% without significantly affecting overall exposure or renal clearance at steady state [99].

At the same time, atorvastatin (OATP1B1 and OATP1B3 substrate; weak CYP3A4 inhibitor), when taken together with edoxaban, does not affect the peak or total exposure of edoxaban [99]. Co-administration of naproxen and edoxaban also had no effect on the peak and total exposure of edoxaban. However, led to an increase in the duration of bleeding compared with each drug administered separately. Co-administration of naproxen increased the baseline-adjusted bleeding time ratio by 72% on day 2 compared with edoxaban alone (90% CI: 139.3–213.3). In contrast, concomitant administration of edoxaban with naproxen increased the equivalent bleeding time by 22% compared with naproxen alone (90% CI: 98.1–151.0) [102]. Naproxen reduced the baseline-adjusted platelet aggregation coefficient on the 2nd day of co-administration by 69.89% (90% CI: 68.20–71.62), while edoxaban itself did not affect platelet aggregation.

Co-administration of high doses of aspirin (325 mg) increased the stationary peak and total exposure of edoxaban by 34% and 30%, respectively, and decreased renal clearance by 17%, possibly due to inhibition of active renal secretion. Co-administration of low-dose aspirin (100 mg) did not affect the peak or total exposure of edoxaban either after a single dose or with stable use (90% CI: 80–125%). Co-administration of edoxaban and aspirin at low (100 mg) or high (325 mg) doses resulted in an additive effect in terms of increased bleeding time. The anticoagulant effects of edoxaban were not affected by the simultaneous administration of aspirin. Coadministration of low doses of aspirin (100 mg) did not significantly affect INR, prothrombin time (PTI), activated partial thromboplastin time (APTT), or intrinsic FXa activity [102]. Enoxaparin did not affect the peak and total exposure of edoxaban with simultaneous dosing or with an interval of 12 hours. Co-administration of edoxaban at a dose of 60 mg and subcutaneous enoxaparin at a dose of 1 mg/kg led to an increase in the effect on the parameters of the analysis of thrombin formation compared to any of the drugs introduced separately. The effect was generally not additive, with the exception of the delay in thrombin formation and the time to peak. The effect on anti-FXa with the simultaneous use of both drugs was additive [103].

Candidate genes influencing the concentration of edoxaban are genes encoding key enzymes of its metabolism: *CES1*, *CYP3A4/5*, *ABCB1* [54] and, to a lesser extent, *SLCO1B1* [104].

Edoxaban and its active metabolite M4 are substrates for P-gp encoded by *ABCB1* (*MDR1*) gene and the organic anion carrier protein OATP1B1 encoded by *SLCO1B1* gene. The pharmacogenomic analysis combined genotype and concentration-time data in 458 healthy volunteers in 14 completed phase 1 studies. The SNVs effect of *ABCB1* gene (rs1045642: C3435T) and *SLCO1B1* gene (rs4149056: T521C) on pharmacokinetic parameters of edoxaban was studied. Although some pharmacological inhibitors of P-gp and OATP1B1 increased exposure to edoxaban, C3435T (rs1045642) of *ABCB1* gene, nor T521C (rs4149056) of *SLCO1B1* gene did not affect the pharmacokinetics of edoxaban. Although, a slight increase in M4 exposure was observed in carriers of minor allele C* of *SLCO1B1* gene [104].

Only a limited amount of edoxaban is metabolized by liver cytochrome P450 isoenzymes (less than 4%) [105]. Metabolites M4 and M1 are formed during the hydrolysis of edoxaban with the participation of the CES1 enzyme encoded by *CES1* gene, while M6 is formed through metabolism with the participation of the CYP3A4/5 isofermet, encoded by *CYP3A5* gene [92]. Analysis of genomic associations showed that SNVs of *CES1* gene affect the plasma levels of dabigatran [106]. So far, no studies have been found on the effect of carriage of the studied SNVs of CES1 gene on the pharmacokinetics of edoxaban. However, this may be promising in terms of personalized selection of DOACs.

There is probably a high risk of developing edoxaban-induced adverse reactions due to a slowdown in the metabolism of the drug in the liver when combined with drug inhibitors of the CYP3A5 isoenzyme in homozygous carriers of non-functional alleles *CYP3A5*. Thus, in patients belonging to the group of non-expressing CYP3A5 (homozygous carriers of the above non-functional alleles), dosing of edoxaban should be calculated with caution and requires monitoring of the risk of bleeding. Co-administration of edoxaban with other drugs metabolized with the participation of the isoenzyme CYP3A5 should be avoided in non-expressors, including antipsychotics (olanzapine), antiestrogens (tamoxifen), antineoplastic (irinotecan, docetaxel, vincristine), immunomodulatory agents (tacrolimus), antiplatelet agents (clopidogrel), antihypertensive agents (nifedipine, amlodipine, felodipine, verapamil), antiviral (indinavir, nelfinavir, ritonavir, saquinavir), HMG-CoA reductase inhibitors (atorvastatin), antibiotics (clarithromycin), steroids (testosterone, estradiol, progesterone and androstenedione), antimalarial drugs (mefloquine, artemether, lumefantrine) [107].

6. Conclusion

The results carried out to the present fundamental and clinical studies of DOACs studies demonstrate an undeniable the influence of genome changes on the pharmacokinetics and pharmacodynamics of DOACs. However, the studies need to be continued. There is a need to plan and conduct larger studies in various ethnic groups with the inclusion of sufficient associative genetic studies of the number of patients in each of the documented groups treatments with well-defined phenotypes. Additional work needed to translation of research results into real clinical practice using results of pharmacogenetic testing and taking into account genomic variations for selection DOACs, their starting and target dosages, which is especially important when the need for long-term pharmacotherapy.

Author details

Natalia Shnayder[1,2*], Marina Petrova[2], Elena Bochanova[1], Olga Zimnitskaya[2], Alina Savinova[2], Elena Pozhilenkova[1] and Regina Nasyrova[2,3]

1 Bekhterev National Medical Research Center of Psychiatry and Neurology (V.M. Bekhterev NMRC PN), St.-Petersburg, Russian Federation

2 Voyno-Yasenetsky Krasnoyarsk State Medical University (V.F. Voyno-Yasenetsky KrasSMU), Krasnoyarsk, Russian Federation

3 Kazan Federal University (KFU), Kazan, Russian Federation

*Address all correspondence to: naschnaider@yandex.ru

References

[1] Heit JA. Venous thromboembolism: disease burden, outcomes and risk factors. J Thromb Haemost. 2005; 3(8):1611-1617. doi: 10.1111/j.1538-7836.2005.01415.x

[2] Feigin VL, Lawes CM, Bennett DA, Barker-Collo SL, Parag V. Worldwide stroke incidence and early case fatality reported in 56 population-based studies: a systematic review. Lancet Neuro.l 2009;8(4):355-369. doi:10.1016/S1474-4422(09)70025-0

[3] Falck-Ytter Y, Francis CW, Johanson NA, Curley C, Dahl OE, SchulmanS, OrtelTL, PaukerS.G., Colwell Jr CW. Prevention of VTE in orthopedic surgery patients: antithrombotic therapy and prevention of thrombosis, 9th ed: American College of chest Physicians evidence-based clinical practice guidelines. Chest. 2012;141(2):e278S; doi:10.1378/chest.11-2404

[4] Pedersen AB, Mehnert F, Sorensen HT, Emmeluth C, Overgaard S, Johnsen S.P. The risk of venous thromboembolism, myocardial infarction, stroke, major bleeding and death in patients undergoing total hip and knee replacement. Bone Joint J. 2014;96:4799-4805; doi:10.1302/0301-620x.96b4.33209

[5] Ezekowitz MD, Bridgers SL, James KE, Carliner NH, Colling CL, Gornick CC, Krause-Steinrauf H, Kurtzke JF, Nazarian SM, Radford MJ, Rickles FR, Shabetai R., Deykin D. Warfarin in the prevention of stroke associated with nonrheumatic atrial fibrillation. Veterans Affairs Stroke Prevention in Nonrheumatic Atrial Fibrillation Investigators. N Engl J Med. 1992; 327(20):1406-1412. Erratum in: N Engl J Med. 1993; 328(2):148. doi: 10.1056/NEJM199211123272002

[6] Simonneau G, Sors H, Charbonnier B, Page Y., Laaban JP, Azarian R, Laurent M, Hirsch JL, Ferrari E, Bosson JL, Mottier D, Beau B. A comparison of low-molecular-weight heparin with unfractionated heparin for acute pulmonary embolism. The THESEE Study Group. Tinzaparine ou Heparine Standard: Evaluations dans l'Embolie Pulmonaire. NEnglJMed. 1997;337(10):663-669. doi: 10.1056/NEJM199709043371002

[7] HolfordNH.Clinicalpharmacokinetics and pharmacodynamics of warfarin. Understanding the dose-effect relationship. Clin Pharmacokinet. 1986;11(6):483-504. doi: 10.2165/00003088-198611060-00005

[8] Shendre A, Parmar GM, Dillon C, Beasley TM, Limdi NA. Influence of age on warfarin dose, anticoagulation control, and risk of hemorrhage. Pharmacotherapy. 2018;38(6):588-596. doi:10.1002/phar.2089

[9] Shatzel JJ, Daughety MM, Prasad V, DeLoughery TG. Reversal of warfarin era thinking. J Intern Med 2018; 283(4):408-410. doi: 10.1111/joim.12697

[10] Barnes GD. Predicting the quality of warfarin therapy: reframing the question. Thromb Haemost. 2019;119(4):509-511. doi: 10.1055/s-0039-1681060

[11] Wu AH. Pharmacogenomic-guided dosing for warfarin: too little too late? Per Med. 2018;15(2):71-73. doi: 10.2217/pme-2017-0080

[12] Schulman S, Kearon C, Kakkar AK, Mismetti P, Schellong S, Eriksson H, Baanstra D, Schnee J, Goldhaber SZ. Dabigatran versus warfarin in the treatment of acute venous thromboembolism. N Engl J Med. 2009; 361(24):2342-2352. doi: 10.1056/NEJMoa0906598

[13] Stangier J, Rathgen K, Stähle H, GansserD, RothW.Thepharmacokinetics,

pharmacodynamics and tolerability of dabigatran etexilate, a new oral direct thrombin inhibitor, in healthy male subjects. Br J Clin Pharmacol. 2007;64(3):292-303. doi: 10.1111/j.1365-2125.2007.02899.x

[14] Hankey GJ, Eikelboom JW. Dabigatran etexilate: a new oral thrombin inhibitor. Circulation. 2011;123(13):1436-50. doi: 10.1161/CIRCULATIONAHA.110.004424

[15] Goldsack NR, Chambers RC, Dabbagh K, Laurent GJ. Thrombin. Int J Biochem Cell Biol. 1998; 30(6):641-646. doi: 10.1016/s1357-2725(98)00011-9

[16] Davie EW, Kulman JD. An overview of the structure and function of thrombin. Semin Thromb Hemost. 2006;32(1):3-15. doi: 10.1055/s-2006-939550

[17] Comin J, Kallmes DF. Dabigatran (Pradaxa). Am J Neuroradiology. 2002; 33(3), 426-428. doi:10.3174/ajnr.a3000

[18] Gelosa P, Castiglioni L, Tenconi M, Baldessin L, Racagni G, Corsini A, Bellosta S. Pharmacokinetic drug interactions of the non-vitamin K antagonist oralanticoagulants (NOACs). Pharmacol Res. 2018;135:60-79. doi:10.1016/j.phrs.2018.07.016

[19] Comuth WJ, Henriksen LØ, van de Kerkhof D, Husted SE, Kristensen SD, de Maat MPM, Münster AMB. Comprehensive characteristics of the anticoagulant activity of dabigatran in relation to its plasma concentration. Thromb Res. 2018;164:32-39. doi: 10.1016/j.thromres.2018.02.141

[20] Antonijevic NM, Zivkovic ID, Jovanovic LM, Matic DM, Kocica MJ, Mrdovic IB , Kanjuh VI, Culafic MD. Dabigatran - metabolism, pharmacologic properties and drug interactions. Curr Drug Metab. 2017;18(7):622-635. doi: 10.2174/1389200218666170427113504

[21] Fawzy AM, Lip GYH. Pharmacokinetics and pharmacodynamics of oral anticoagulants used in atrial fibrillation. Expert Opin Drug Metab Toxicol. 2019;15(5):381-398. doi: 10.1080/17425255.2019.1604686

[22] Satoh T, Hosokawa M. Structure, function and regulation of carboxylesterases. Chem Biol Interact. 2006;162(3):195-211. doi: 10.1016/j.cbi.2006.07.001

[23] Ghosh S., Natarajan R. Cloning of the humanc holesterylesterhydrolase promoter: identification of functional peroxisomal proliferator-activate drecept or responsive elements. Biochem Biophys Res Commun. 2001;284(4):1065-1070. doi: 10.1006/bbrc.2001.5078

[24] Shi J, Wang X, Nguyen JH, Bleske BE, Liang Y, Liu L, Zhu HJ. Dabigatran etexilate activation is affected by the CES1 genetic polymorphism G143E (rs71647871) and gender. Biochem Pharmacol. 2016;119:76-84. doi:10.1016/j.bcp.2016.09.003

[25] Chen Z, Shi T, Zhang L, Zhu P, Deng M, Huang C, Hu T, Jiang L, Li J. Mammalian drug efflux transporters of the ATP binding cassette (ABC) family in multidrug resistance: A review of the past decade. Cancer Let.t 2016;370(1):153-164. doi: 10.1016/j.canlet.2015.10.010

[26] Gouin-Thibault I, Delavenne X, Blanchard A, Siguret V, Salem JE, Narjoz C, Gaussem P, Beaune P, Funck-Brentano C, Azizi M, Mismetti P, Loriot MA. Interindividual variability in dabigatran and rivaroxaban exposure: contribution of ABCB1 genetic polymorphisms and interaction with clarithromycin. J Thromb Haemost.

2017; 15(2):273-283. doi: 10.1111/jth.13577

[27] Bernier M, Lancrerot SL, Rocher F, Van-Obberghen EK, Olivier P, Lavrut T, Parassol-Girard N, Drici MD. Major bleeding events in octagenarians associated with drug interactions between dabigatran and P-gp inhibitors. J Geriatr Cardiol. 2019; 16(11):806-811. doi: 10.11909/j.issn.1671-5411.2019.11.002

[28] Daud ANA, Bergman JEH, Bakker MK, Wang H, Kerstjens-Frederikse WS, de Walle HEK, Groen H, Bos JHJ, Hak E, Wilffert B. P-Glycoprotein-mediated drug interactions in pregnancy and changes in the risk of congenital anomalies: a case-reference study. Drug Saf. 2015; 38(7):651-659. doi: 10.007/s40264-015-0299-3

[29] Ebner T, Wagner K, Wienen W. Dabigatran acylglucuronide, the major human metabolite of dabigatran: in vitro formation, stability, and pharmacological activity. Drug Metab Dispos 2010; 38(9):1567-1575. doi: 10.1124/dmd.110.033696

[30] UniProt. UDP-glucuronosyltransferase 2B15. UniProt Knowledgebase. www.uniprot.org/uniprot/P54855. April 22 2020

[31] Chung JY, Cho JY, Yu KS, Kim JR, Jung HR, Lim KS, Jang IJ, Shin SG. Effect of the UGT2B15 genotype on the pharmacokinetics, pharmacodynamics, and drug interactions of intravenous lorazepam in healthy volunteers. Clin Pharmacol Ther. 2005;77(6):486-494. doi:10.1016/j.clpt.2005.02.006

[32] Paré G, Eriksson N, Lehr T, Connolly S, Eikelboom J, Ezekowitz MD, Axelsson T, Haertter S, Oldgren J, Reilly P, Siegbahn A, Syvanen AC, Wadelius C, Wadelius M, Zimdahl-Gelling H, Yusuf S, Wallentin L. Genetic determinants of dabigatran plasma levels and their relation to bleeding. Circulation. 2013;127(13):1404-1412. doi: 10.1161/CIRCULATIONAHA

[33] Dimatteo C, D'Andrea G, Vecchione G, Paoletti O, Cappucci F, Tiscia GL, Buono M, Grandone E, Testa S, Margaglione M. Pharmacogenetics of dabigatran etexilate interindividual variability. Thromb Res. 2016; 144:1-5. doi:10.1016/j.thromres.2016.05.025

[34] He X., Hesse L.M., Hazarika S., Masse G, Harmatz JS, Greenblatt DJ, Court MH. Evidence for oxazepam as an in vivo probe of UGT2B15: oxazepam clearance is reduced by UGT2B15 D85Y polymorphism but unaffected by UGT2B17 deletion. Br J Clin Pharmacol. 2009;68(5):721-730. doi: 10.1111/j.1365-2125.2009.03519.x

[35] Court MH, Zhu Z, Masse G, Duan SX, James LP, Harmatz JS, Greenblatt DJ. Race, gender, and genetic polymorphism contribute to variability in acetaminophen pharmacokinetics, metabolism, and protein-adduct concentrations in healthy African-American and European-American volunteers. J Pharmacol Exp Ther. 2017;362(3):431-440. doi: 10.1124/jpet.117.242107

[36] Savelyeva MI, Urvantseva IA, Ignatova AK, Panchenko JS, Poddubnaya IV. Pharmacogenetic features of the phase II biotransformation of tamoxifen: a systematic review. Pharmacogenetics and Pharmacogenomics. 2017;(1):10-15. (In Russ.)

[37] Ethell BT, Anderson GD, Burchell B. The effect of valproic acid on drug and steroid glucuronidation by expressed human UDP-glucuronosyltransferases. Biochem Pharmacol. 2003;65(9):1441-1449. doi: 10.1016/s0006-2952(03)00076-5

[38] Stringer F, Ploeger BA, DeJongh J, et al. Evaluation of the impact of UGT polymorphism on the pharmacokinetics

and pharmacodynamics of the novel PPAR agonist sipoglitazar. J Clin Pharmacol. 2013;53(3):256-263. doi: 10.1177/0091270012447121

[39] Perzborn E, Roehrig S, Straub A, Kubitza D, Mueck W, Laux V. Rivaroxaban: a new oral Factor Xa inhibitor. Arterioscler Thromb Vasc Biol. 2010;30:376-381. doi: 10.1161/ATVBAHA.110.202978

[40] Turpie AGG. Oral, direct Factor Xa inhibitors in development for the prevention and treatment of thromboembolic diseases. Arterioscler Thromb Vasc Biol. 2007;27:1238-1247. doi: 10.1161/ATVBAHA.107.139402

[41] Kubitza D, Becka M, Voith B, Zuehlsdorf M, Wensing G. Safety, pharmacodynamics, and pharmacokinetics of single doses of BAY 59-7939, an oral, direct factor Xa inhibitor. Clin Pharmacol Ther. 2005;78(4):412-421. doi: 10.1016/j.clpt.2005.06.011,

[42] Kubitza D, Becka M, Wensing G, Voith B, Zuehlsdorf M. Safety, pharmacodynamics, and pharmacokinetics of BAY 59-7939--an oral, direct Factor Xa inhibitor--after multiple dosing in healthy male subjects. Eur J Clin Pharmacol. 2005;61(12):873-880. doi: 10.1007/s00228-005-0043-5

[43] Weinz C, Buetehorn U, Daehler HP, Kohlsdorfer C, Pleiss U, Sandmann S, Schlemmer KH, Schwarz T, Steinke W. Pharmacokinetics of BAY 59-7939--an oral, direct Factor Xa inhibitor--in rats and dogs. Xenobiotica. 2005;35(9):891-910. doi: 10.1080/00498250500250493

[44] Weinz C, Schwarz T, Kubitza D, Mueck W, Lang D. Metabolism and excretion of rivaroxaban, an oral, direct factor Xa inhibitor, in rats, dogs, and humans. Drug Metab Dispos. 2009;37(5):1056-64. doi: 10.1124/dmd.108.025569

[45] https://www.ema.europa.eu/en/documents/assessment-report/xarelto-epar-public-assessment-report_en.pdf

[46] Mueck W., Kubitza D., Becka M. Co-administration of rivaroxaban with drugs that share its elimination pathways: pharmacokinetic effects in healthy subjects. Br J Clin Pharmacol. 2013;76(3):455-466. doi: 10.1111/bcp.12075

[47] Xie Q, Xiang Q, Mu G, Ma L, Chen S, Zhou S, Hu K, Zhang Z, Cui Y, Jiang J. Effect of *ABCB1* genotypes on the pharmacokinetics and clinical outcomes of new oral anticoagulants: a systematic review and meta-analysis. Current Pharmaceutical Design. 2018;24(30):3558-3565. doi: 10.2174/1381612824666181018153641

[48] Sychev D, Minnigulov R, Bochkov P, Ryzhikova K, Yudina I, Lychagin A, Morozova T. Effect of CYP3A4, CYP3A5, ABCB1 gene polymorphisms on rivaroxaban pharmacokinetics in patients undergoing total hip and knee replacement surgery high. Blood Press Cardiovasc Prev. 2019;26(5):413-420. doi: 10.1007/s40292-019-00342-4

[49] Sennesael A-L, Panin N, Vancraeynest C, Pochet L, Spinewine A, Haufroid V, Elens L. Effect of ABCB1 genetic polymorphisms on the transport of rivaroxaban in HEK293 recombinant cell lines. Sci Rep. 2018;8(1):10514. doi: 10.1038/s41598-018-28622-4

[50] Kanuri SH, Kreutz RP. Pharmacogenomics of novel direct oral anticoagulants: newly identified genes and genetic variants. J Pers Med. 2019;9(1):7. doi: 10.3390/jpm9010007

[51] Cusatis G, Sparreboom A. Pharmacogenomic importance of ABCG2. Pharmacogenomics. 2008;9(8):1005-1009. doi: 10.2217/14622416.9.8.1005

[52] Cusatis G, Gregorc V, Li J, Spreafico A, Ingersoll RG, Verweij J, Ludovini V,

Villa E, Hidalgo M, Sparreboom A, Baker SD. Pharmacogenetics of ABCG2 and adverse reactions to gefitinib. J Natl Cancer Inst. 2006;98(23):1739-1742. doi: 10.1093/jnci/djj469

[53] Woodward OM, Tukaye DN, Cui J, Greenwell P, Constantoulakis LM, Parker BS, Rao A, Köttgen M, Maloney PC, Guggino WB. Gout-causing Q141K mutation in ABCG2 leads to instability of the nucleotide-binding domain and can be corrected with small molecules. Proc Natl Acad Sci U S A. 2013;110(13):5223-5228. doi: 10.1073/pnas.1214530110

[54] O'Connor CT, Kiernan TJ, Yan BP. The genetic basis of antiplatelet and anticoagulant therapy: A pharmacogenetic review of newer antiplatelets (clopidogrel, prasugrel and ticagrelor) and antico-agulants (dabigatran, rivaroxaban, apixaban and edoxaban). Expert Opin Drug Metab Toxicol. 2017;13(7):725-739. doi: 10.1080/17425255.2017.1338274

[55] Solus JF, Arietta BJ, Harris JR, Sexton DP, Steward JQ, McMunn C, Ihrie P, Mehall JM, Edwards TL, Dawson EP. Genetic variation in eleven phase I drug metabolism genes in an ethnically diverse population. Pharmacogenomics. 2004;5(7):895-931. doi: 10.1517/14622416.5.7.895

[56] Galgani A, Palleria C, Iannone LF, De Sarro G, Giorgi FS, Maschio M, Russo E. Pharmacokinetic interactions of clinical interest between direct oral anticoagulants and antiepileptic drugs. Front Neurol. 2018;9:1067. doi: 10.3389/fneur.2018.01067

[57] Brings A, Lehmann M-L, Foerster KI, Burhenne J, Weiss J, Haefeli WE, Czock D. Perpetrator effects of ciclosporin (P-glycoprotein inhibitor) and its combination with fluconazole (CYP3A inhibitor) on the pharmacokinetics of rivaroxaban in healthy volunteers. Br J Clin Pharmacol. 2019;85(7):1528-1537. doi: 10.1111/bcp.13934

[58] Harskamp RE, Teichert M, Lucassen WAM, van Weert HCPM, Lopes RD. Impact of polypharmacy and P-glycoprotein- and CYP3A4-modulating drugs on safety and efficacy of oral anticoagulation therapy in patients with atrial fibrillation. Cardiovasc Drugs Ther. 2019;33(5):615-623. doi: 10.1007/s10557-019-06907-8

[59] Wu SN, Zhang Y, Gardner CO, Chen Q, Li Y, Wang GL, Gao PJ, Zhu DL. Evidence for association of polymorphisms in CYP2J2 and susceptibility to essential hypertension. Ann Hum Genet. 2007;71(4):519-525. doi: 10.1111/j.1469-1809.2007.00346.x

[60] Luettgen JM, Knabb RM, He K, Pinto DJ, Rendina AR. Apixaban inhibition of factor Xa: Micro-scopic rate constants and inhibition mechanism in purified protein systems and in human plasma. J Enzyme Inhib Med Chem. 2011;26(4):514-526. doi: 10.3109/14756366.2010.535793

[61] Ansell J. Factor Xa or thrombin: is factor Xa a better target? J Thromb Haemost. 2007;5(1):60-64. doi: 10.1111/j.1538-7836.2007.02473.x

[62] Jiang X, Crain EJ, Luettgen JM, Schumacher WA, Wong PC. Apixaban, an oral direct factor Xa inhibitor, inhibits hu-man clot-bound factor Xa activity in vitro. Thromb Haemost. 2009;101(4):780-782. doi: 10.1160/th08-07-0486

[63] Savinova AV, Petrova MM, Shnayder NA, Bochanova EN, Nasyrova RF. Pharmacokinetics and pharmacogenetics of apixaban. Rational Pharmacotherapy in Cardiology. 2020;16(5):852-860. (In Russ.). doi:10.20996/1819-6446-2020-10-17

[64] Byon W, Nepal S, Schuster AE, Shenker A, Frost CE.

Regional gastrointestinal absorption of apixaban in healthy subjects. J Clin Pharmacol. 2018;58(7):965-971. doi: 10.1002/jcph.1097

[65] Vakkalagadda B, Frost C, Byon W, Boyd RA, Wang J, Zhang D, Yu Z, Dias C, Shenker A, LaCreta F. Effect of rifampin on the pharmacokinetics of apixaban, an oral direct inhibitor of factor Xa. Am J Cardiovasc Drugs. 2016;16(2):119-127. doi: 10.1007/s40256-015-0157-9

[66] Raghavan N, Frost CE, Yu Z, He K, Zhang H, Humphreys WG, Pinto D, Chen S, Bonacorsi S, Wong PC, Zhang D. Apixaban metabolism and pharmacokinetics after oral administration to humans. Drug Metab Dispos. 2009;37(1):74-81. doi: 10.1124/dmd.108.023143

[67] Wang L, Zhang D, Raghavan N, Yao M, Ma L, Frost CE, Maxwell BD, Chen S, He K, Goosen TC, Humphreys WG, Grossman SJ. In vitro assessment of metabolic drug-drug interaction po-tential of apixaban through cytochrome P450 phenotyping, inhibition, and induction studies. Drug Metab Dispos. 2010;38(3):448-458. doi: 10.1124/dmd.109.029694

[68] Zhang D, He K, Herbst JJ, Kolb J, Shou W, Wang L, Balimane PV, Han YH, Gan J, Frost CE, Humphreys WG. Characterization of efflux transporters involved in distribution and disposition of apixaban. Drug Metab Dispos. 2013;41(4):827-835. doi: 10.1124/dmd.112.050260

[69] Frost C, Wang J, Nepal S, Schuster A, Barrett YC, Mosqueda-Garcia R, Reeves RA, LaCreta F. Apixaban, an oral, direct factor Xa inhibitor: single dose safety, pharmacokinetics, pharmacodynamics and food effect in healthy subjects. Br J Clin Pharmacol. 2013;75(2):476-487. doi: 10.1111/j.1365-2125.2012.04369.x

[70] Frost C, Nepal S, Wang J, Schuster A, Byon W, Boyd RA, Yu Z, Shenker A, Barrett YC, Mosqueda-Garcia R, Lacreta F. Safety, pharmacokineticsandpharmacodynamics of multiple oral doses of apixaban, a factor Xa inhibitor, in healthy subjects. Br J Clin Pharmacol. 2013;76(5):776-786. doi: 10.1111/bcp.12106

[71] He K, Luettgen JM, Zhang D, He B, Grace Jr JE, Xin B, Pinto DJP, Wong PC, Knabb RM, Lam PYS, Wexler RR, Grossman SJ. Preclinical pharmacokineticsandpharmacodynamics of apix-aban, a potent and selective factor Xa inhibitor. Eur J Drug Metab Pharmacokinet. 2011;36(3):129-139. doi: 10.1007/s13318-011-0037-x

[72] Wang X, Mondal S, Wang J, Tirucherai G, Zhang D, Boyd RA, Frost C. Effect of activated charcoal on apixaban pharmacokinetics in healthy subjects. Am J Cardiovasc Drugs. 2014;14(2):147-154. doi: 10.1007/s40256-013-0055-y

[73] Ueshima S, Hira D, Fujii R, Kimura Y, Tomitsuka C, Yamane T, Tabuchi Y, Ozawa T, Itoh H, Horie M, Terada T, Katsura T. Impact of ABCB1, ABCG2, and CYP3A5 polymorphisms on plasma trough concentrations of apixaban in Japanese patients with atrial fibrillation. Pharmacogenet Genomics. 2017;27(9):329-336. doi: 10.1097/FPC.0000000000000294

[74] SNPedia. CYP3A5. Accessed October 20, 2020. https://www.snpedia.com/index.php/CYP3A5

[75] Kang RH, Jung SM, Kim KA, Lee DK, Cho HK, Jung BJ, Kim YK, Kim SH, Han C, Lee MS, Park JY. Effects of CYP2D6 and CYP3A5 genotypes on the plasma concentrations of risperidone and 9-hydroxyrisperidone in Korean schizophrenic patients. J Clin Psychopharmacol. 2009;29(3):272-7. doi: 10.1097/JCP.0b013e3181a289e0

[76] Canonico M, Bouaziz E, Carcaillon L, Verstuyft C, Guiochon-Mantel A, Becquemont L, Scarabin PY. Synergism between oral estrogen therapy and cyto-chrome P450 3A5*1 allele on the risk of venous thromboembolism among postmenopausal women. J Clin Endocrinol Metab. 2008;93(8):3082-3087. doi: 10.1210/jc.2008-0450

[77] SNPedia. CYP1A2. https://www.snpedia.com/index.php/CYP1A2. Access date: September 19 2020

[78] Sri H, Kanuri SH, Kreutz RP. Pharmacogenomics of novel direct oral anticoagulants: newly identi-fied genes and genetic variants. J Pers Med. 2019;9(1):7. doi: 10.3390/jpm9010007

[79] Sweezy T, Mousa SA. Genotype-guided use of oral antithrombotic therapy: A pharmacoeconomic perspective. Pers. Med. 2014;11:223-235. doi: 10.2217/pme.13.106

[80] Carlini EJ, Raftogianis RB, Wood TC, Jin F, Zheng W, RebbeckTR,WeinshilboumRM.Sulfation pharmacogenetics: SULT1A1 and SULT1A2 allele frequencies in Caucasian, Chinese and African-American subjects. Pharmacogenetics. 2001;11:57-68. doi: 10.1097/00008571-200102000-00007

[81] Wang L, Raghavan N, He K, Luettgen JM, Humphreys WG, Knabb RM, Pinto DJ, Zhang D. Sulfation of o-demethyl apixaban: enzyme identification and species comparison. Drug Metab. Dispos. 2009;37:802-808. doi: 10.1124/dmd.108.025593

[82] Nagar S, Walther S, Blanchard RL. Sulfotransferase (SULT) 1A1 polymorphic variants *1, *2, and *3 are associated with altered enzymatic activity, cellular phenotype, and protein degradation. Mol. Pharmacol. 2006;69:2084-2092. doi: 10.1124/mol.105.019240

[83] Raftogianis RB, Wood TC, Otterness DM, Van Loon JA, Weinshilboum R.M. Phenol sulfotransferase pharmacogenetics in humans: association of common SULT1A1 alleles with TS PST phenotype. Biochem. Biophys. Res. Commun. 1997;239:298-304. doi: 10.1006/bbrc.1997.7466

[84] Fuji T, Fujita S, Kawai Y, Nakamura M, Kimura T, Fukuzawa M, Abe K, Tachibana S. Efficacy and safety of edoxaban versus enoxaparin for the prevention of venous thromboembolism following total hip arthroplasty: STARS J-V. Thromb J. 2015;13:27. doi: 10.1186/s12959-015-0057-x

[85] Fuji T, Wang CJ, Fujita S, Kawai Y, Kimura T, Tachibana S. Safety and efficacy of edoxaban, an oral factor Xa inhibitor, for thromboprophylaxis after total hip arthroplasty in Japan and Taiwan. J Arthroplasty. 2014;29(12):2439-2446. doi: 10.1016/j.arth.2014.05.029

[86] Fuji T, Fujita S, Kawai Y, Nakamura M, Kimura T, Kiuchi Y, Abe K, Tachibana S. Safety and ef-ficacy of edoxaban in patients undergoing hip fracture surgery. Thromb Res. 2014;133(6):1016-1022. doi: 10.1016/j.thromres.2014.03.009

[87] Samama MM, Mendell J, Guinet C, Le Flem L, Kunitada S. In vitro study of the anticoagulant effects of edoxaban and its effect on thrombin generation in comparison to fondaparinux. Thromb Res. 2012;129(4):e77-82. doi: 10.1016/j.thromres.2011.07.026

[88] Ogata K, Mendell-Harary J, Tachibana M, Masumoto H, Oguma T, Kojima M, Kunitada S. Clini-cal safety, tolerability, pharmacokinetics, and pharmacodynamics of the novel factor Xa inhibitor edoxaban in healthy volunteers. J Clin Pharmacol. 2010;50(7):743-53. doi: 10.1177/0091270009351883

[89] Matsushima N, Lee F, Sato T, Weiss D, Mendell J. Bioavailability and safety of the Factor Xa inhibitor edoxaban and the effects of quinidine in healthy subjects. Clin Pharmacol Drug Dev. 2013;2(4):358-366. doi: 10.1002/cpdd.53

[90] Parasrampuria DA, Kanamaru T, Connor A, Wilding I, Ogata K, Shimoto Y, Kunitada S. Evalua-tion of regional gastrointestinal absorption of edoxaban using the enterion capsule. J Clin Pharmacol. 2015;55(11):1286-1292. doi: 10.1002/jcph.540

[91] Parasrampuria DA, Truitt KE. Pharmacokinetics and pharmacodynamics of edoxaban, a non-vitamin K antagonist oral anticoagulant that inhibits clotting Factor Xa. Clin Pharmacokinet. 2016;55(6):641-655. doi: 10.1007/s40262-015-0342-7

[92] Bathala MS, Masumoto H, Oguma T, He L, Lowrie C, Mendell J. Pharmacokinetics, biotransfor-mation, and mass balance of edoxaban, a selective, direct factor Xa inhibitor, in humans. Drug Metab Dispos. 2012;40(12):2250-2255. doi: 10.1124/dmd.112.046888

[93] Sankyo D. Inc. Savaysa (edoxaban tosylate): FDA Cardiovascular and Renal Drugs Adviso-ry Committee briefing document. NDA 206316. Accessed October 20, 2020. http://www.fda.gov/AdvisoryCommittees/CommitteesMeetingMaterials/Drugs/CardiovascularandRenalDrugsAdvisoryCommittee/ucm420703.htm

[94] Jönsson S, Simonsson US, Miller R, Karlsson MO. Population pharmacokinetics of edoxaban and its main metabolite in a dedicated renal impairment study. J Clin Pharmacol. 2015;55(11):1268-1279. doi: 10.1002/jcph.541

[95] Mikkaichi T, Yoshigae Y, Masumoto H, Imaoka T, Rozehnal V, Fischer T, Okudaira N, Izumi T. Edoxaban transport via P-glycoprotein is a key factor for the drug's disposition. Drug Metab Dis-pos. 2014;42(4):520-528. doi: 10.1124/dmd.113.054866

[96] FDA Center for Drug Evaluation Research. FDA draft guidance for industry: drug interaction studies—study design, data analysis, implications for dosing, and labeling recommendations. Accessed October 20, 2020. http://www.fda.gov/downloads/Drugs/Guidances/ucm292362.pdf,

[97] Flockhart D.A. Drug interactions: cytochrome P450 drug interaction table. Indiana University School of Medicine. Accessed October 20, 2020. https://static.medicine.iupui.edu/divisions/clinpharm/content/p450_Table_Oct_11_2009.pdf

[98] Parasrampuria DA, Mendell J, Shi M, Matsushima N, Zahir H, Truitt K. Edoxaban drug-drug in-teractions with ketoconazole, erythromycin, and cyclosporine. Br J Clin Pharmacol. 2016;82(6):1591-1600. doi: 10.1111/bcp.13092

[99] Mendell J, Zahir H, Matsushima N, Noveck R, Lee F, Chen S, Zhang G, Shi M. Drug-drug inter-action studies of cardiovascular drugs involving P-glycoprotein, an efflux transporter, on the pharmacokinetics of edoxaban, an oral factor Xa inhibitor. Am J Cardiovasc Drugs. 2013;13(5):331-342. doi: 10.1007/s40256-013-0029-0

[100] Cordarone® (amiodarone HCl) tablets: full prescribing information. Wyeth Pharmaceuticals Inc., a subsidiary of Pfizer Inc.; Philadelphia. Accessed October 20, 2020. http://labeling.pfizer.com/showlabeling.aspx?id=93

[101] Mendell J, Chen S, He L, Desai M, Parasramupria DA. The effect of rifampin on the pharmaco-kinetics

of edoxaban in healthy adults. Clin Drug Investig. 2015;35(7):447-453. doi: 10.1007/s40261-015-0298-2

[102] Mendell J, Lee F, Chen S, Worland V, Shi M, Samama MM. The effects of the antiplatelet agents, aspirin and naproxen, on pharmacokinetics and pharmacodynamics of the anticoagulant edoxaban, a direct factor Xa inhibitor. J Cardiovasc Pharmacol. 2013;62(2):212-221. doi: 10.1097/FJC.0b013e3182970991

[103] Zahir H, Matsushima N, Halim AB, He L, Zhang G, Lee F, Worland V, Mendell J. Edoxaban administration following enoxaparin: a pharmacodynamic, pharmacokinetic, and tolerability as-sessment in human subjects. Thromb Haemost. 2012;108(1):166-175. doi: 10.1160/TH11-09-0676

[104] Vandell AG, Lee J, Shi M, Rubets I, Brown KS, Walker JR. An integrated pharmacokinet-ic/pharmacogenomic analysis of ABCB1 and SLCO1B1 polymorphisms on edoxaban exposure. Pharmacogenomics J. 2018;18(1):153-159. doi: 10.1038/tpj.2016.82

[105] Bounameaux H, Camm AJ. Edoxaban: an update on the new oral direct factor Xa inhibitor. Drugs. 2014;74(11):1209-1231. doi: 10.1007/s40265-014-0261-1. Erratum in: Drugs. 2014;74(12):1455 DOI: 10.1007/s40265-014-0261-1

[106] StangierJ.Clinicalpharmacokinetics and pharmacodynamics of the oral direct thrombin inhibitor dabigatran etexilate. Clin Pharmacokinet. 2008;47(5):285-295. doi: 10.2165/00003088-200847050-00001

[107] Umamaheswaran G, Kumar DK, Adithan C. Distribution of genetic polymorphisms of genes en-coding drug metabolizing enzymes & drug transporters - a review with Indian perspective. Indian J Med Res. 2014;139(1):27-65.

Chapter 6

Possibilities of Combinatorial Therapy: Insulin Dysregulation and the Growth Hormone Perspective on Neurodegeneration

Priyanka Sengupta and Debashis Mukhopadhyay

Abstract

RTKs have been reported to be implicated in several neurodegenerative disorders and the roles of insulin receptor family have emerged as a key common pathway across diseases. Thus we focussed on the Insulin receptor family and discussed the irregulation from the growth hormone axis. The signaling, regulation and physiology of the production in liver and CNS has never been discussed in signaling perspectives and is extremely crucial for understanding the possibilities of IGF1 in neurodegeneration specifically. The commonalities across neurodegenerative diseases such as oxidative stress, mitochondrial dysfunction, and protein misfolding and insulin pathway anomalies have been elucidated and correlated with the insulin pathway. The crosstalk possibilities of the pathways, along with other regulatory modes for the development of combinatorial therapy have been discussed to visualize a common platform for neurodegenerative diseases including AD, PD, HD, ALS and FTD. Furthermore, the incretin based therapies that have gradually emerged as alternatives for insulin based therapy due to its inherent drawback of resistance has been briefly discussed.

Keywords: neurodegeneration, insulin, IGF1, GPCR, combinatorial therapy, lncRNA, Alzheimer's disease

1. Introduction

Insulin dysregulation is a common phenomenon in several diseases, though their cause-effect relationship with progression is debatable. This review focuses on the degenerative pathways but essentially incorporates cues from proliferative mechanisms to develop a holistic approach towards understanding the disease progression. In case of neurodegeneration such as that in Alzheimer's disease [AD], Huntington disease [HD], Fronto temporal Dementia [FTD] and Parkinson's disease [PD], insulin dysregulation has been reported [1]. Therapies have been successfully developed encompassing the insulin pathway in ADwhere intranasal administration of insulin assists in recuperation, however resistance towards insulin and mode of administration remains an elusive matter [2]. Similar strategies are gradually being developed for FTD as well using Novolin-R insulin [3]. Insulin shock therapy for the schizophrenic patients was one of the initial approaches towards tackling the disease, but with time insulin resistance or insensitivity to higher dosages led to search for better ways of ameliorating the disease on relapse [4]. Insulin like growth factor 1 [IGF1] therapy has been implemented in ADbut due to the lack of conclusive evidence, resistance and contentious results from experimental models, the attempt did not stand the test of time [5]. It is thus impending to further investigate the modes of regulation and pathways which could lead the therapeutic development.

Insulin receptor family is a subset of the broader Receptor Tyrosine kinase [RTK] family comprised of 20 precise receptor sub-families further sub divided into more families based on ligand and domains of the receptors that play varied roles in neurodegeneration [6]. They include ErbB, PDGF, Ins, VEGF, FGF, Trk, PTK7, Ror, MuSK, Met, Axl, Tie, Eph, Ret, Ryk, DDR, ROS, LMR, STYK1 and ALK [7]. Many of these families have been shown to be involved in AD, PD as well as proliferative diseases such as cancer. The alterations in expression as well as activity has been documented which clearly elucidates the importance of understanding the roles of these receptors in disease pathology. With respect to neurodegeneration however, the roles played by RTKs are gradually being explored and understood since the complexities both on the membrane front and intracellular pathways are numerous. Insulin receptor family composed of Insulin Receptor [INSR], Insulin like growth factor receptor [IGF1R, IGF2R], and Insulin receptor related receptor [INSRR] [8] forms a common bridge for understanding neurodegenerative pathways as they are implicated in almost all diseases and relatively well studied yet poorly understood. It is crucial to mention that unlike other members of the insulin family, INSRR is an orphan receptor with no known ligand. Recent studies have shown that it is pH sensitive and the receptor is activated by alkaline pH [9]. IGF2R unlike IGF1R is non-mitogenic and involved in targeting IGF2 to lysosomes for degradation. It basically functions in signal attenuation and on overexpression has been reported to increase the amyloid beta generation [10].

Thus we begin with an overview of the hallmarks of neurodegeneration, their underlying mechanisms in brief and then delve into the possibility of therapeutics encompassing insulin pathway as a future prospect for palliation of neurodegeneration. Insulin pathway involves mainly insulin andIGF1 which elicit different roles in the cell despite being structurally similar with common pathways that had been studied for decades but is still poorly understood in the context of neurodegeneration. Insulin pathway being a metabolic pathway primarily, is capable of modulating several downstream important signaling molecules and influences metabolism, growth and survival through P13K pathway and MAPK mediated pathway that determines cellular fate [11]. IGF1 additionally engages in the Jak–stat pathway [12] and uses several components of the GPCR pathways and in turn get regulated by them as well [13].

2. Commonalities of neurodegenerative diseases

Neurodegenerative diseases like Alzheimer's and Parkinson have been long studied and the key proteins identified have been tried and tested for targeting in order to ameliorate the disease. However most of it has failed [14]. Several mutations have been identified for both such as *APOEε*4 allele, APP, PSEN1 and PSEN2 for AD, but people without any of these mutations have also been found to develop the disease [15], which adds to the complexity. The triggers for both these diseases have been shown to be associated with multiple factors as diverse as gut microbiota for PD [16], bacterial infections of the gum for AD [17], or genetic pre disposition and epigenetic modifications.

Patients with Huntington often develop diabetes, whereas those with diabetes are more prone to developing AD [18]. The impairment of insulin pathways is common across patients suffering from different neurodegenerative diseases. Studies with transfected striatal nerve cells in vitro, showed that IGF1 can block the mutant protein huntingtin-induced cellular death and decreases formation of intranuclear inclusions [19]. Reduction in apoptosis was perhaps not the reason for this observation since BDNF which does the same, did not prohibit formation of such inclusions. The mitochondrial dysfunction in these striatal cell lines derived from huntingtin Knock-in mice is perhaps ameliorated by insulin and IGF1. The roles of these factors have further been observed in several studies where reduced energy metabolism in lymphoblasts derived from HD patients was shown to be associated with downregulation of Akt and Erk activation which can be helped with IGF1 and insulin [20].

ALS and FTD are different diseases but both elicit a degeneration of neurons, their clinical as well as pathological manifestations are similar. Interestingly both of these display alterations in Growth hormone and IGF1 secretions [21]. ALS was initially characterized by the mutation in a gene, Superoxide dismutase [SOD1] with a 10–20% incidence in patients and since then more than a hundred different types of SOD1 mutations that cause ALS has been discovered [22]. The trigger for ALS and proposed mechanism though could be through growth hormones anomaly, could as well be through glutamate-induced neurotoxicity with an aberrant increase in glutamate concentration in CSF [23].

The aggregated proteins form intra cellular inclusions or extra cellular aggregates in different brain areas. These proteins usually have a beta -sheet structure that allows aggregation and fibril formation as part of the misfolding process [24]. Misfolding of protein aggregates is one of the key underlying cause of neurodegeneration. Amyloid fibrils form plaques found in AD, Phosphorylated tau leads to neurofibrillary tangles, prions mediate in neurodegeneration and alpha synuclein aggregates in PD are also common [25].

In case of PD, ALS and AD, upto10% cases are inherited. However, in HD almost every case has a familial history [26]. The common disease/common variant [CD/CV] hypothesis explains that common disorders are governed by common DNA variants which elevates risks but are usually not causative factors and might add to the understanding of genetic involvement in phenotypic manifestation of disease [27]. For example, the Apolipoprotein E [APOE] encodes a 299 amino acid long glycoprotein and is estimated to be a major contributing factor in AD development. It has also been reported in PD [27]. This similarity further elicits that neurodegenerative disorders might have a common underlying protein–protein interaction network (**Figure 1**). Also, intervention for neurodegenerative disorders could be facilitated by exploring the genes and its regulatory components including ncRNAs that might govern the progression and allow scope of regulating the protein–protein network downstream [28, 29]. Studies have focused on individual disorders but rarely generated a common platform that allows better understanding of the network by taking varied disorders into perspective.

Amongst the hallmarks of neurodegeneration that significantly contributes towards the progression is oxidative stress. It has been implicated in several diseases, including AD, PD and ALS [30]. Extensive oxidation of lipids, DNA and proteins leads to deactivation of major processes or upregulation of toxic cellular cascades. The imbalance in the scales of Reactive oxygen species [ROS] generation damages the cells [31]. Amyloid beta which is originally generated by neurons in AD in response to insults and cellular damage in pursuit of protection, in turn coordinates iron and copper to generate peroxide that accelerates ROS generation by Fenton chemistry [14]. Dopamine buildup in cytoplasm in PD coordinates iron and induces ROS formation. Active site destabilization of SOD also allows further oxidation. Such unregulated

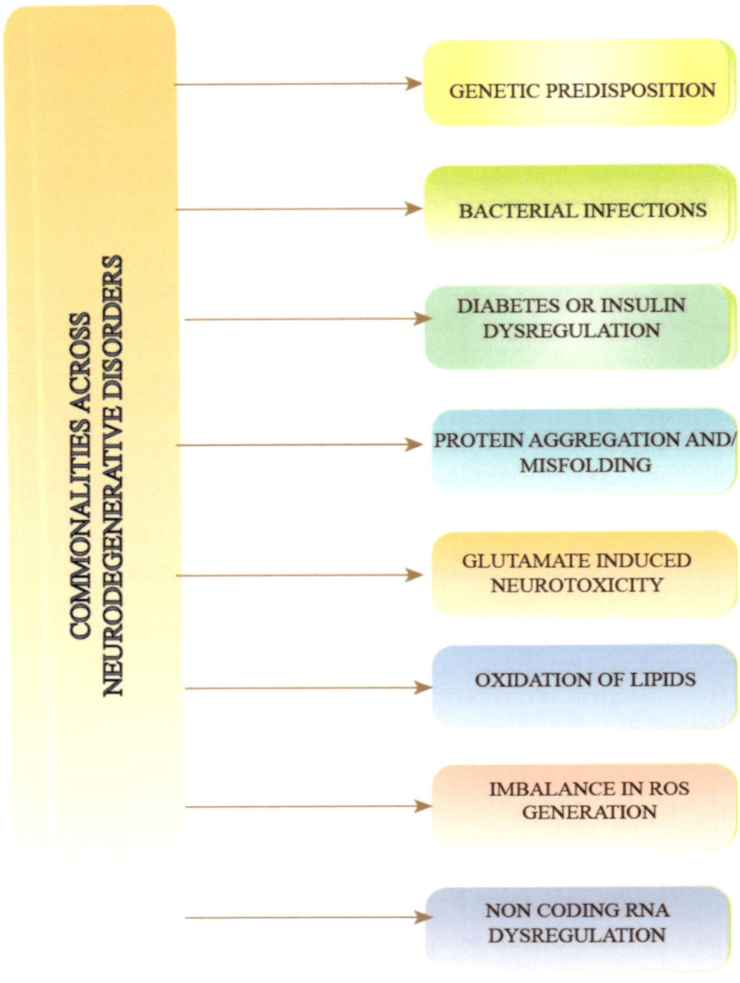

Figure 1.
Commonalities across neurodegenerative disorders, two or more are often shared.

ROS further affects calcium regulation which leads to excitotoxicity [32]. The current drugs encompassing ROS generation affect the rate of progression at late stages and thus it is increasingly important to understand the growth hormone axis that changes early in the disease cycle and determines the final outcome, ROS generation and toxic misfolding of proteins aggregates amongst other catastrophic events that lay ahead of the domino like cascade of neurodegenerative pathways.

3. Insulin resistance and neuroinflammation

The growth factors bind to receptors and they no longer respond to the ligand binding when resistance develops, which would have otherwise triggered a cascade of downstream signaling. Several studies have attempted to evaluate the total IGF1 or Insulin levels that are responsible for the resistance to overcome it. Dosage up to 100 nM Insulin even instead of physiologically relevant 1 nM have been unsuccessful in reinstating the sensitivity. This further drives attention towards the receptor [33]. The anomalies in the reports pertaining to the receptor stimulation particularly in AD clearly elucidate a faulty signaling cascade operating at different stages of the disease [2]. The receptors of the Insulin family, vis-à-vis INSR and IGF1R are elusive and bind to both ligands, Insulin and IGFs. Their diverse intracellular domains allows them to bind several other adaptor proteins other than the conventional mediators of signaling cascade, IRS1 and IRS2 [34]. There are numerous astounding facts about these receptors which make them unique targets and add to their therapeutic value. INSR and IGF1R forms hybrids that has a higher affinity for IGF1 [35–37] but their activity if its varied from individual dimers and their respective localization after stimulation is unknown. The insulin resistance poses a major setback to its therapeutic value and correcting the axis by identifying other players in the cascade both downstream and at the membrane front could thus help in re-sensitizing the receptors.

Both Insulin and IGF1R has been shown to enter the nucleus when activated recently and it is speculated that they perform physiological roles which might be altered in different disease situations [38]. It has been experimentally illustrated as an orchestrated event that occurs physiologically in non-cancerous cell lines along with different cancers, in which this behavior of nuclear migration was first found. It however remains due to illustrate the proportions of the nuclear and cytoplasmic amount of IGF1R in different disease conditions where these metabolic signaling pathways are known to be altered. Their phosphorylation status too remains to be explored since IGF1R has multiple phosphorylation sites [39] and they could be important in understanding their role in neurodegeneration.

Recent studies show that phosphoINSR can be translocated into the nucleus in a clathrin mediated manner. It forms a complex with RNA pol-II, HCF 1 and DNA binding transcription factors like THAP 11. Mass-spectrometry data shows the translocation involves KPNA 2 and HSP 70 [40].

IGF-1R has been observed in the nucleus in case of prostate cancer and breast cancer cells. Full length IGF-1R alpha and beta chains were reported in the nuclear extract of prostate cancer cells. This is the only example of a receptor which traffics as individual sub unit to the nucleus [41]. Other RTKs such EGFR, FGFR has also been previously been observed in the nucleus. The endocytosis is here both clathrin and caveolin mediated. The nuclear transport here is not mediated by adaptor proteins like IRS 1 or an inherent NLS but by SUMOylation [42].

The cause and effect relationship for the ever so complex pathway and its involvement in AD or PD remains unclear and further experimental studies are required to investigate the connection of this underlying nuclear migration with disease progression. The ligands and receptors need to betreated an individual elements instead of a holistic component in the cascade, since there remains the possibility that Insulin and IGF1 both can stimulate other receptors [43]. The concerned receptors could be activated in diseases like AD by Amyloid beta fragments [44, 45] and behave differently in terms of interacting partners and localization, thus altering the signaling cascade majorly.

4. Insulin as a growth factor with prospects in therapeutics for neurodegeneration

Insulin production in the body was assumed to primarily happen in the pancreas and circulated throughout, however production in the CNS of both insulin and IGF1 is now proven [46–48]. Insulin production in CNS appears to be important for the lower organisms than that in higher organism like humans. However further research in the last decade has yielded results that clearly indicate that insulin is secreted in the CNS and might play important roles in physiology. The amount of the same is presumed to be lower compared to the pancreas derived insulin which is transported into the brain through receptor mediated transcytosis. However it can also be independent of the receptor as illustrated by [49]. Insulin circulating in the bloodstream binds to receptors present on the endothelial cells at the blood brain barrier which is further moved into the interstitial fluid. There it binds to insulin receptors distributed throughout the cerebral cortex, olfactory bulb, hippocampus, hypothalamus, amygdala and septum [48]. IGF1 on the other hand, binds to one of its 6 binding proteins and remains in the inactive form in the bloodstream and in local tissues. The entrance into the brain occurs in a similar fashion as in the case of insulin [50].

Several parts of the brain are sensitive towards insulin and they have a different relationship associated with the alterations of the levels. Neuroimaging studies have shed light on the insulin induced brain responses in the fusiform gyrus, hippocampus, pre-frontal cortex, striatum, hypothalamus and insular cortex. Thus healthy insulin signaling controls brain networks implicated in reward processing, memory retrieval, homeostatic control and cognitive control in general [51]. These wide involvements of insulin in regulation of distinct parts of the brain responsible for different activities leads to the marked impact of a mild dysregulation and thus indicate an alteration could infact be an initial event in the cascade of neurodegeneration.

Insulin is known to activate cell growth, cell repair, mitochondrial activity, gene expression, energy utilization and protein synthesis for decades. In both AD and PD, insulin signaling pathway and downstream regulators contribute significantly to the pathology of the disease. Insulin signaling in the brain of these patients is desensitized and while analyzing post-mortem brains, it appears that they have inactivated receptors and downstream IRS1 and 2 as well. The key secondary messengers of this signaling pathway, Akt and mTOR also appears to be inactivated in these patients as it is observed diabetes [14, 20, 27]. Thus, AD was termed as Type 3 diabetes where a systemic resistance to the pathway occurs [52]. However, unlike diabetes the reasons could be very different. Insulin desensitization occurring in the brain could be part and parcel of the inflammatory response in the brain. In case of AD, where amyloid beta aggregates lead to plaque formation, the oxidative stress and cytokines involvement in the long run could restrict the supply of the insulin and IGF essential for growth and repair of the neurons [53]. Pro-inflammatory cytokines like Tumor necrosis factor [TNF] could possibly block the signaling pathways of insulin and IGF1.

Saenger et al. [54] investigated into the SOD1-G93A mouse lines that elicit ALS like pathology, both mild and severe phenotype form. The results indicated IGF1 therapy in the early stages can be effective but in case of severe cases, the functional outcomes were no better. Despite increase signaling in brain, at high doses, survival chances did not improve. Clinical trials that evaluated the role of Growth hormones in patients with ALS yielded mixed results. Researchers back in 1993 employed a very small dosage [0.1 mg/day] which impacted the IGF1 levels after therapy. In another study recently in 2012, 2.8 mg/day was used, but that further led to a reduction in the IGF1 and IGF1-BP3 demonstrating the effectiveness of the therapy further [46].

5. IGF1 as a pleiotropic factor in aging and neurodegeneration

The brain receives its IGF1 supply through both autocrine and paracrine pathways. IGF1 is secreted by liver, in response to binding of growth hormone [GH] to their respective GH receptors, which leads to increase in the circulating IGF1 levels. The IGF1 thus secreted by liver then binds to their receptors IGF1R in the pituitary and hypothalamus, which in turn inhibits Growth hormone releasing hormone [GHRH] and Growth hormone [GH] production [46].

The hepatic IGF1 production makes up for 70% of the total circulating ligand pool and caters to the brain by passing through the blood brain barrier at choroid plexus directly into the Cerebrospinal fluid [CSF] with the assistance of IGF1R and Megalin, a low density lipoprotein receptor related protein 2 transporter [46]. There is a clear feedback loop for the hepatic production regulation, but not for the autocrine production in the brain (**Figure 2**). Studies show mutations that manifest in GH deficiency or resistance present normal cognitive functionality [55] however when IGF1 production is globally eradicated or insensitivity is induced, that leads to microcephaly and cognitive deficits in children [56]. This suggests the autocrine brain production might be preserved in GH mutated scenarios and a separate feedback loop exists for that regulation. Adding to the complexity, the circulated IGF1 is bound to IGF binding proteins [IGFBPs] mainly IGFBP-3 being the most abundant, making them unavailable for receptor stimulation [57].

The autocrine production though expected to be independent of the hepatic IGF1 production, appears to decline with age similarly. The endocrine decline in IGF1 levels has been related to the diminished GH pulse frequency and amplitude, observed in case of aging. It is partly due to the decrease in ghrelin binding to GH secretagogue receptor [GHSR] [57]. Aging and lowering of cognitive abilities is observed to be associated with lower levels of IGF1, where the receptor levels increase to compensate

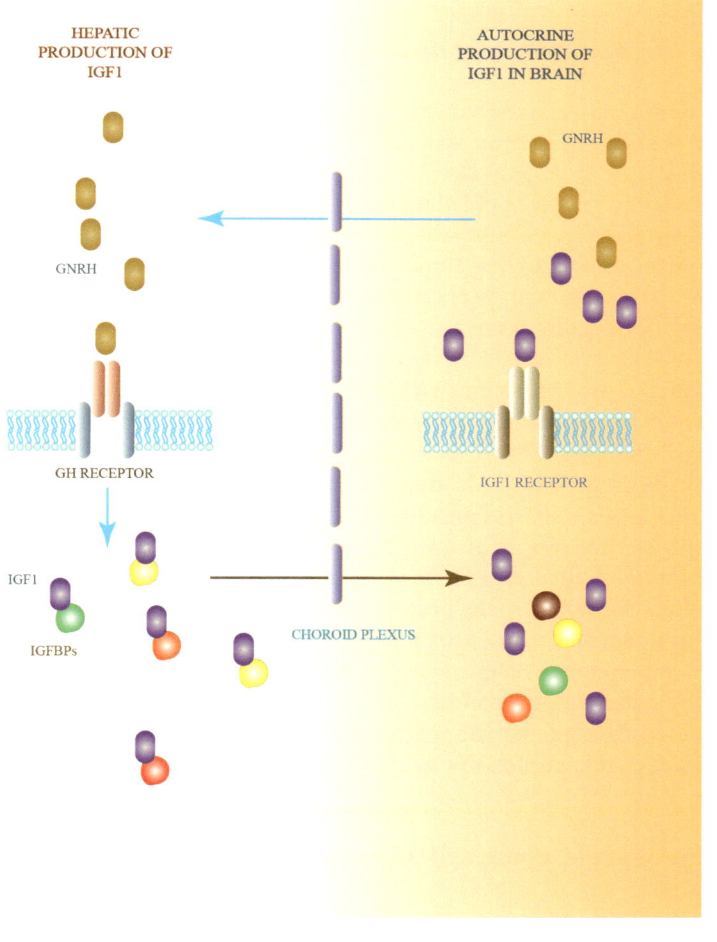

Figure 2.
Feedback loop for hepatic and autocrine production of IGF1 in the brain.

for the lower availability perhaps. The increase in the receptor levels in aged individuals could also be a coping mechanism for combating insults and stress induced due to the breach in blood brain barrier. Nevertheless, it is evident that IGF1 plays a major neutrophic role within PNS and CNS and is strongly involved in neurogenesis, anti-apoptotic, synaptogenesis and anti-inflammatory effects at cortical, sensory and motor levels and hence further investigation into the puzzling characteristics of the receptor shall shed light on the definitive involvement in neurodegeneration.

IGF1 other than being implicated in AD and other neurodegenerative diseases is also a major risk factor for cancer. Its upregulation is a major implication of proliferation in several cancers. Modulation of the cell cycle, apoptosis and cell survival through interaction with IRS1 and IRS2 and downstream effectors like PI3K/AKT/mTOR allows IGF1 to drive the cell towards proliferation [58]. Some pre-clinical studies state that mutations in genes that control the GF/INS/IGF axis can increase the lifespan even in invertebrate and vertebrate animal models [59].

Aging and IGF1 are intertwined on several levels, adding to the complexity of the insulin pathway. Research shows IGF1 deficiency could slower aging [60–63] and thus is a separate concern for therapy development for patients who develop Late onset AD [LOAD]. However combinatorial treatment with other membrane receptor antagonists or agonists for that matter which are implicated in the diseases could offer better options for prophylaxis.

6. Impact of growth factors on the neurophysiology

The amyloid hypothesis that focuses primarily on the protein misfolding that occurs in AD and aggregation associated with it largely fails at analyzing the actual neuronal pathophysiological developments in the brain. Inflammatory mediators like cytokines can promote the state in CNS through several mechanisms, crossing the BBB or entering by circumventricular organs, communication transmitted via the vagal nerve, and signaling through the cerebral endothelium [51]. These pathways allow insinuation and perpetuation of pro-inflammatory responses within the brain. Amyloid beta oligomerisation and tau phosphorylation which are hallmarks of AD can also be promoted through such changes [51].

The impact of growth factors comes into play since important cellular phenomena like inflammation and underlying reasons for neuronal loss are in turn corrected with insulin based therapies. The problems with such therapies persist, and have been long known, as progressive resistance. Key growth factors present in the brain such as BDNF, NGF, GDNF, IGF1 and insulin all lose their capacity of reversing or controlling the damage over time [64]. However, the improvements are often long lasting and disease progression is halted effectively by them through receptors in the glia initially [51]. Neurodegenerationis a complex process andfactors like GLP1, GIP1, and insulin cross the blood brain barrier in order to provide protection on several levels including ROS generation. In response to these, synaptic activity as well as plasticity is restored, brain functionality and memory retention is improved, and mitogenesis and mitochondrial function which dysregulates the energy utilization is also corrected [65]. Autophagy occurs normally and apoptosis rates are reduced as well.

7. Future prospects: cross talk between insulin signaling and other pathways

In order to improve the capabilities of the insulin therapy and circumvent the issues with hyperinsulinemia, it is important to understand the crosstalk possibilities for this important axis. The goal to re-sensitize the cells towards treatment or induce a similar cascade by receptor stimulation through other ligands or adaptors could pave the way for combinatorial therapy. Thus, understanding the cross talk possibilities for neurodegenerationis impending. In case of heart diseases a crosstalk between insulin receptors and beta 2 adrenergic receptors [β_2AR] is found which paved the path towards understanding the exploitation of GPCR signaling pathways by RTKs [66]. RTKs can use Beta arrestin, G protein receptor kinases, insulin to directly induce tissue RAS activation, regulate beta-adrenergic catecholamine stimulation and even to attenuate contractile response to β_2AR stimulation in myocardial ischemia [67].

Angiotensin II [AII] acts on the cell by virtue of its receptor and since 1996, the direct connection between the two pathways on the phosphorylation and the downstream P13K activity has been known. Stimulation with AII inhibited both basal and insulin stimulated PI3K activity in rats [68].

Amongst interesting findings, IGF1R has been found to exist in association with $GABA_B$, which offers neuroprotection to cerebellar granule neurons from low potassium induced apoptosis. This process involves Akt recruitment and activation of IGF1R with the assistance of $G_{i/o}$- protein and FAK1 [69, 70]. Antidepressants can potentially trans-activate RTKs like EGFR by inducing activation of LPA receptors [71]. Reports show that acute MOR agonists can induce beta arrestin dependent and src-dependent IGF1R transactivation through subsequent Erk phosphorylation, prolonged treatment with the agonist however leads to heterologous desensitization of IGF1R based cascade [72]. The studies corroboratively indicate insulin GPCR heterocomplex plays important roles in different tissues and several of such associations could be involved in neurons in physiological and disease scenarios as well.

Studies show IGF1 receptor signaling and anti-apoptotic activity in cortical neurons is partly due to the Src dependent PACAP type I receptor which is transactivated [73]. Non-canonical insulin pathway receptors like TrkA has also been observed in such complexes with another receptor LPA1 that allows for constitutive activation of the cascade involving ERK1/2 in response to NGF [71]. IGF1 can also mediate G protein dependent ERK1/2 activation through transactivation of sphingosine 1 phosphate receptors [73].

Dopamine and Insulin signaling pathways are also intertwined as they elicit a reciprocal relationship. Antagonism of D2 receptors for a short duration leads to upregulation of insulin secretion [74]. Insulin can also enhance reuptake of dopamine, which has been visualized with respect to mental health and metabolic syndromes.

Recent studies on ncRNAs are also evolving and shows that several lnc RNAs and miRs that are involved in controlling key phenomena in neurodegenerative diseases like AD, PD, HD and ALS. Long non-coding RNAs like BACE1-AS, XIST are upregulated in AD [75, 76]. Neat1 and MALAT1 are upregulated in FTD as well as ALS, where they form paraspeckles with TDP-43 and FUS proteins. UCHL1-AS1 leads to perturbation of ubiquitin-proteasome system that and is upregulated in PD. HTT-AS, HAR1 and BDNF-AS were reported to be dysregulated in HD. Interestingly, insulin responsiveness of these genes have not been explored in neuronal perspective. Some lncRNAs such as H19, lncASIR have been reported by several groups [29, 77] but their implications and involvement, interaction with other proteins or ncRNAs shall open up avenues for therapy oriented research. Furthermore, Lnc RNAs that are known to interact with these receptors such as IRAIN, GAS5, NNT-AS1 [78] needs to be studied in the neurodegenerative landscape to allow translational medicine development.

8. Combinatorial and peptide based therapies: insulins, incretins and drugs

Insulin resistance remains a major challenge towards drug development and meanwhile alternative strategies encompassing hormones are being tested and developed forneurodegenerative diseases. Incretin hormones like GLP1 and GIP show similar therapeutic roles and do not lead to insulin desensitization, as they do not activate the receptors however they lend similar effects [79]. Furthermore, analogues of the peptide hormones do not affect the blood glucose levels in non-diabetics with normoglycemic index. The side effects are mild loss of appetite and nausea. Detemir study led to this important realization that drugs for non-diabetic with AD or PD who require intervention with hormones needs to be developed with caution. Those with higher peripheral insulin resistance performed better with the drug, however those with lower peripheral resistance suffered from worsening of memory formation. Though there is plenty to understand and explore about the insulin pathway and its role in complex multifactorial neurodegenerative diseases, the treatments encompassing these factors that appears to be effective must be discussed.

GLP1 is part of a peptide based growth factor family that activates a glucagon type GPCR, expressed in primates, rodents and human neurons. Other receptor agonists such as lixisenatidemliraglutide and semaglutide available for treating Type II diabetes are also being tested for eeffectiveness in AD and PD [1]. Some of them can traverse the blood brain barriers and are thus prospective game changers for therapeutics. GLP 1 mimetic have shown promising results in animal models of AD, they exhibit fascinating reduction of chronic inflammation which is a major driver for progression of disease.

GIP is another sister incretin that bind to a GPCR on the membrane and its receptor is abundant in a wide range of cells including pyramidal neurons, Purkinje cells in cerebellum and basal brain areas. It was capable of offering neuroprotection to APP/PS1 mice, reduced loss of synapses and recreated synaptic plasticity [79]. Furthermore, the amyloid plaque load was also reduced along with oxidative stress and DNA damage.

9. Conclusions

Substantial advancement in the field of growth hormone, RTKs and their involvement in neurodegeneration has been made in the last two decades. The development of peptide based therapies involving incretins that can mitigate the degenerative processes in the brain is a major feat that shows promise. Controlling this major InsR and IGF1R, which are prominent and one of the most important albeit in age reversal [61, 80] is yet to be achieved but picking up cues from diseases like cancer that elicits an alternate pathway [81], in terms of therapy could accelerate the process of developing therapies (**Figure 3**). The ability of growth factors to modulate cellular events such as ROS generation, energy utilization and others are remarkable and thus developing more sophisticated approaches using the knowledge thus gathered to invoke the right set of signals for slowing the cycle and early detection are important. Though possibilities involving the insulin pathway have been only explored on the protein level, regulation on the RNA level could be utilized yet to enhance sensitivity.

Pre-clinical studies from growth hormone therapies often leave out important aspects like multiple binding partners, transactivation and cross talks that leads to different results when applied to humans. Research on analogues with no resistance, compounds that re-instate sensitivity and alternative drugs such as mAbs against

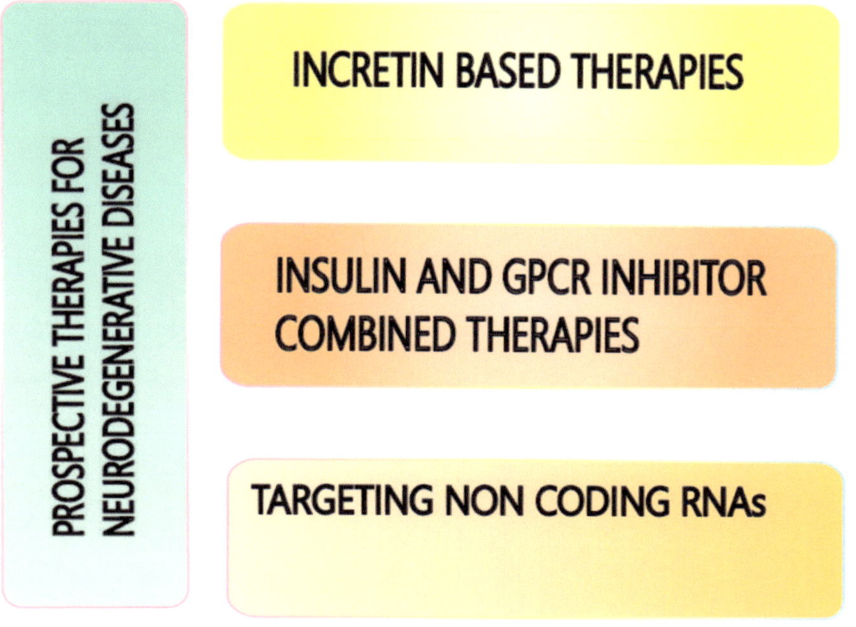

Figure 3.
Therapies that could exploit the unified approach and yield therapeutic benefits.

RTKs altered are the need for the hour. The current peptide based drugs on the market are promising since they can potentially reverse a range of pathophysiological parameters of neurodegeneration. However understanding the hormonal axis that led to the death is important for further biomarker development and therapy development as well. The growth hormone axis could indeed be an underlying cause amongst the plethora of factors already known for neurodegeneration. Studies on their involvement in determining cellular fate and their tuning in accordance with progression of disease are required for developing a better understanding about stages of the progressive disorders discussed holistically. The crosstalk with other pathways and gradual involvement of several miR and Lnc RNA which are crucial are complicating the story and yet simplifying it in terms of the puzzling and contentious results.

In conclusion, it is apparent that the neurodegenerative disorders have an underlying insulin pathway abnormality and growth hormone axis plays a major role the CNS and in turn affects progression of neurodegeneration. The Insulin receptor family amongst the RTKs is an important set that could lead the path towards therapies for degenerative disorders in a non-invasive manner if understood in their entirety and the regulation though complex could be a common network of protein–protein interaction that would simplify prognosis and prophylaxis.

Acknowledgements

We would like to acknowledge Dr. DebdattoMookherjee, Universität Basel for his constant motivation and constructive feedback during manuscript preparation.

Conflict of interest

The authors declare no conflict of interest.

Author details

Priyanka Sengupta and Debashis Mukhopadhyay*
Biophysics and Structural Genomics Division, Saha Institute of Nuclear Physics, Homi Bhabha National Institute, Kolkata, India

*Address all correspondence to: debashis.mukhopadhyay@saha.ac.in

References

[1] Hölscher C. Brain insulin resistance: role in neurodegenerative disease and potential for targeting. Expert Opin Investig Drugs [Internet]. 2020;29[4]:333-48. Available from: https://doi.org/10.1080/13543784.2020.1738383

[2] Kim B, Elzinga SE, Henn RE, McGinley LM, Feldman EL. The effects of insulin and insulin-like growth factor I on amyloid precursor protein phosphorylation in in vitro and in vivo models of Alzheimer's disease. Neurobiol Dis. 2019 Dec 1;132:104541.

[3] Rosenbloom MH. Intranasal Insulin in Frontotemporal Dementia [FTD] - Full Text View - ClinicalTrials.gov [Internet]. 2020 [cited 2021 Feb 4]. Available from: https://clinicaltrials.gov/ct2/show/NCT04115384

[4] Agarwal SM, Caravaggio F, Costa-Dookhan KA, Castellani L, Kowalchuk C, Asgariroozbehani R, et al. Brain insulin action in schizophrenia: Something borrowed and something new. Neuropharmacology. 2020;163[May].

[5] Bianchi VE, Locatelli V, Rizzi L. Neurotrophic and neuroregenerative effects of GH/IGF1. Int J Mol Sci. 2017;18[11]:1-25.

[6] Majumder P, Roy K, Bagh S, Mukhopadhyay D. Receptor tyrosine kinases [RTKs] consociate in regulatory clusters in Alzheimer's disease and type 2 diabetes. Mol Cell Biochem [Internet]. 2019;459[1-2]:171-82. Available from: https://doi.org/10.1007/s11010-019-03560-5

[7] Shpakov AO, Derkach K V., Berstein LM. Brain signaling systems in the Type 2 diabetes and metabolic syndrome: Promising target to treat and prevent these diseases. Futur Sci OA. 2015;1[3].

[8] Haeusler RA, McGraw TE, Accili D. Metabolic Signalling: Biochemical and cellular properties of insulin receptor signalling. Nat Rev Mol Cell Biol [Internet]. 2018;19[1]:31-44. Available from: http://dx.doi.org/10.1038/nrm.2017.89

[9] Deyev IE, Popova N V., Serova O V., Zhenilo S V., Regoli M, Bertelli E, et al. Alkaline pH induces IRR-mediated phosphorylation of IRS-1 and actin cytoskeleton remodeling in a pancreatic beta cell line. Biochimie [Internet]. 2017;138:62-9. Available from: http://dx.doi.org/10.1016/j.biochi.2017.04.002

[10] Lewitt MS, Boyd GW. The Role of Insulin-Like Growth Factors and Insulin-Like Growth Factor–Binding Proteins in the Nervous System. Biochem Insights. 2019;12:117862641984217.

[11] Katsel P, Roussos P, Beeri MS, Gama-Sosa MA, Gandy S, Khan S, et al. Parahippocampal gyrus expression of endothelial and insulin receptor signaling pathway genes is modulated by Alzheimer's disease and normalized by treatment with anti-diabetic agents. PLoS One. 2018;13[11]:1-18.

[12] Zhu S, Mohammed Soutto, Zheng Chen, M. Blanca Piazuelo, M. Kay Washington, Abbes Belkhiri, Alexander Zaika DP& WE-R. Activation of IGF1R by DARPP-32 promotes STAT3 signaling in gastric cancer cells. Oncogene. 2019;38:5805-5816.

[13] Suleymanova N, Crudden C, Shibano T, Worrall C, Oprea I, Tica A, et al. Functional antagonism of β-arrestin isoforms balance IGF-1R expression and signalling with distinct cancer-related biological outcomes. Oncogene [Internet]. 2017;36[41]:5734-44. Available from: http://dx.doi.org/10.1038/onc.2017.179

[14] De La Monte SM, Tong M, Schiano I, Didsbury J. Improved Brain Insulin/IGF Signaling and Reduced Neuroinflammation with T3D-959 in an Experimental Model of Sporadic Alzheimer's Disease. J Alzheimer's Dis [Internet]. 2017 [cited 2021 Feb 4];55[2]:849-64.

[15] Bellenguez C, Grenier-Boley B, Lambert JC. Genetics of Alzheimer's disease: where we are, and where we are going. Curr Opin Neurobiol. 2020;61:40-8.

[16] Hopfner F, Künstner A, Müller SH, Künzel S, Zeuner KE, Margraf NG, et al. Gut microbiota in Parkinson disease in a northern German cohort. Brain Res [Internet]. 2017;1667:41-5. Available from: http://dx.doi.org/10.1016/j.brainres.2017.04.019

[17] Maurer K, Rahming S, Prvulovic D. Dental health in advanced age and Alzheimer's Disease: A possible link with bacterial toxins entering the brain? Psychiatry Res - Neuroimaging [Internet]. 2018;282:132-3. Available from: https://doi.org/10.1016/j.pscychresns.2018.06.009

[18] Shieh JCC, Huang PT, Lin YF. Alzheimer's Disease and Diabetes: Insulin Signaling as the Bridge Linking Two Pathologies. Mol Neurobiol. 2020;57[4]:1966-77.

[19] Bano D, Zanetti F, Mende Y, Nicotera P. Neurodegenerative processes in Huntington's disease. Cell Death Dis. 2011;2[11]:1-7.

[20] Naia L, Ferreira IL, Cunha-Oliveira T, Duarte AI, Ribeiro M, Rosenstock TR, et al. Activation of IGF-1 and Insulin Signaling Pathways Ameliorate Mitochondrial Function and Energy Metabolism in Huntington's Disease Human Lymphoblasts. Mol Neurobiol. 2014;51[1]:331-48.

[21] Suzuki K, Suzuki S, Ishii Y, Fujita H, Matsubara T, Okamura M, et al. Serum insulin-like growth factor-1 levels in neurodegenerative diseases. Acta Neurol Scand. 2019;139[6]:563-7.

[22] Harms MB, Baloh RH. Clinical Neurogenetics: Amyotrophic Lateral Sclerosis. Neurol Clin. 2013;31[4]:929-50.

[23] Spalloni A, Nutini M, Longone P. Role of the N-methyl-d-aspartate receptors complex in amyotrophic lateral sclerosis. Vol. 1832, Biochimica et Biophysica Acta - Molecular Basis of Disease. Elsevier; 2013. p. 312-22.

[24] Interaction of the N -AcA β [13-23] NH 2 Segment Of the Beta Amyloid Peptide with Beta-Sheet-Blocking Peptides: Site and Edge Specificity Banafsheh Mehrazma, Anahit Petoyan, Stanley K. A. Opare, and Arvi Rauk*. :1-28.

[25] Davis AA, Leyns CEG, Holtzman DM. Intercellular Sp read of Protein Aggregates in Neurodegenerative Disease. Annu Rev Cell Dev Biol. 2018;34[July]:545-68.

[26] Ajroud-Driss S, Siddique T. Sporadic and hereditary amyotrophic lateral sclerosis [ALS]. Vol. 1852, Biochimica et Biophysica Acta - Molecular Basis of Disease. Elsevier; 2015. p. 679-84.

[27] Ahmad K, Baig MH, Mushtaq G, Kamal MA, Greig NH, Choi I. Commonalities in Biological Pathways, Genetics, and Cellular Mechanism between Alzheimer Disease and Other Neurodegenerative Diseases: An In Silico-Updated Overview. Curr Alzheimer Res. 2017;14[11]:1190-7.

[28] Wang DQ, Fu P, Yao C, Zhu LS, Hou TY, Chen JG, et al. Long Non-coding RNAs, Novel Culprits, or Bodyguards in Neurodegenerative Diseases. Mol Ther - Nucleic Acids [Internet]. 2018;10[March]:269-76. Available from: https://doi.org/10.1016/j.omtn.2017.12.011

[29] Geng T, Liu Y, Xu Y, Jiang Y, Zhang N, Wang Z, et al. H19 lncRNA promotes skeletal muscle insulin sensitivity in part by targeting AMPK. Diabetes. 2018;67[11]:2183-98.

[30] Picca A, Calvani R, Coelho-Júnior HJ, Landi F, Bernabei R, Marzetti E. Mitochondrial dysfunction, oxidative stress, and neuroinflammation: Intertwined roads to neurodegeneration. Antioxidants. 2020;9[8]:1-21.

[31] Limongi D, Baldelli S. Redox Imbalance and Viral Infections in Neurodegenerative Diseases. Oxid Med Cell Longev. 2016;2016.

[32] Burbulla LF, Song P, Mazzulli JR, Zampese E, Wong YC, Jeon S, et al. Dopamine oxidation mediates mitochondrial and lysosomal dysfunction in Parkinson's disease. Science [80-]. 2017;357[6357]:1255-61.

[33] Talbot K, Wang H-Y, Kazi H, Han L-Y, Bakshi K, Stucky A, et al. Demonstrated brain insulin resistance in Alzheimer's disease patients is associated with IGF-1 resistance, IRS-1 dysregulation, and cognitive decline. J Clin Invest. 2012;122[4]:1316-38.

[34] Lizcano JM, Alessi DR. The insulin signalling pathway. Current biology. 2002 Apr 2;12(7):R236-8

[35] Denley A, Brierley G V., Carroll JM, Lindenberg A, Booker GW, Cosgrove LJ, et al. Differential activation of insulin receptor isoforms by insulin-like growth factors is determined by the C domain. Endocrinology. 2006 Feb;147[2]:1029-36.

[36] Andersen M, Nørgaard-Pedersen D, Brandt J, Pettersson I, Slaaby R. IGF1 and IGF2 specificities to the two insulin receptor isoforms are determined by insulin receptor amino acid 718. PLoS One [Internet]. 2017 Jun 1 [cited 2021 Feb 4];12[6].

[37] Cieniewicz AM, Cooper PR, McGehee J, Lingham RB, Kihm AJ. Novel method demonstrates differential ligand activation and phosphatase-mediated deactivation of insulin receptor tyrosine-specific phosphorylation. Cell Signal. 2016 Aug 1;28[8]:1037-47.

[38] Kesten D, Horovitz-Fried M, Brutman-Barazani T, Sampson SR. Insulin-induced translocation of IR to the nucleus in insulin responsive cells requires a nuclear translocation sequence. Biochim Biophys Acta - Mol Cell Res [Internet]. 2018;1865[4]:551-9. Available from: https://doi.org/10.1016/j.bbamcr.2018.01.004

[39] Kelly GM, Buckley DA, Kiely PA, Adams DR, O'Connor R. Serine phosphorylation of the insulin-like growth factor I [IGF-1] receptor C-terminal tail restrains kinase activity and cell growth. J Biol Chem [Internet]. 2012 Aug 10 [cited 2021 Feb 4];287[33]:28180-94.

[40] Batista TM, Cederquist CT, Kahn CR. The insulin receptor goes nuclear. Cell Res [Internet]. 2019;29[7]:509-11. Available from: http://dx.doi.org/10.1038/s41422-019-0185-0

[41] Aleksic T, Chitnis MM, Perestenko O V., Gao S, Thomas PH, Turner GD, et al. Type 1 insulin-like growth factor receptor translocates to the nucleus of human tumor cells. Cancer Res. 2010;70[16]:6412-9.

[42] Solomon-Zemler R, Sarfstein R, Werner H. Nuclear insulin-like growth factor-1 receptor [IGF1R] displays proliferative and regulatory activities in non-malignant cells. PLoS One. 2017;12[9]:1-14.

[43] Geetha T, Rege SD, Mathews SE, Meakin SO, White MF, Babu JR. Nerve growth factor receptor TrkA, a new

receptor in insulin signaling pathway in PC12 cells. J Biol Chem. 2013;288[33]:23807-13.

[44] Xie L, Helmerhorst E, Taddei K, Plewright B, Van Bronswijk W, Martins R. Alzheimer's beta-amyloid peptides compete for insulin binding to the insulin receptor. J Neurosci. 2002;22[10]:1-5.

[45] Zimbone S, Monaco I, Gianì F, Pandini G, Copani AG, Giuffrida ML, et al. Amyloid Beta monomers regulate cyclic adenosine monophosphate response element binding protein functions by activating type-1 insulin-like growth factor receptors in neuronal cells. Aging Cell. 2018;17[1]:1-10.

[46] Gubbi S, Quipildor GF, Barzilai N, Huffman DM, Milman S. 40 years of IGF1: IGF1: The Jekyll and Hyde of the aging brain. J Mol Endocrinol. 2018;61[1]:T171-85.

[47] Bianchi V, Locatelli V, Rizzi L. Neurotrophic and Neuroregenerative Effects of GH/IGF1. Int J Mol Sci [Internet]. 2017 Nov 17 [cited 2021 Feb 4];18[11]:2441. Available from: http://www.mdpi.com/1422-0067/18/11/2441

[48] Pomytkin I, Costa-Nunes JP, Kasatkin V, Veniaminova E, Demchenko A, Lyundup A, et al. Insulin receptor in the brain: Mechanisms of activation and the role in the CNS pathology and treatment. CNS Neurosci Ther. 2018;24[9]:763-74.

[49] Rhea EM, Rask-Madsen C, Banks WA. Insulin transport across the blood–brain barrier can occur independently of the insulin receptor. J Physiol. 2018;596[19]:4753-65.

[50] Hakuno F, Takahashi S-I. IGF1 receptor signaling pathways. J Mol Endocrinol [Internet]. 2018;61[1]:T69-86. Available from: https://pubmed.ncbi.nlm.nih.gov/29535161/%0Ahttps://jme.bioscientifica.com/view/journals/jme/61/1/JME-17-0311.xml%0Ahttp://www.ncbi.nlm.nih.gov/pubmed/29535161

[51] Kullmann S, Heni M, Hallschmid M, Fritsche A, Preissl H, Häring HU. Brain insulin resistance at the crossroads of metabolic and cognitive disorders in humans. Physiol Rev. 2016;96[4]:1169-209.

[52] Rad SK, Arya A, Karimian H, Madhavan P, Rizwan F, Koshy S, et al. Mechanism involved in insulin resistance via accumulation of β-amyloid and neurofibrillary tangles: Link between type 2 diabetes and alzheimer's disease. Drug Des Devel Ther. 2018;12:3999-4021.

[53] George S Bloom, John S Lazo AN. Reduced brain insulin signaling: A seminal process in Alzheimer's disease pathogenesis. Neuropharmacology [Internet]. 2018;[1;136[Pt B]]:192-5. Available from: https://www.sciencedirect.com/science/article/abs/pii/S0028390817304331

[54] Saenger S, Holtmann B, Nilges MR, Schroeder S, Hoeflich A, Kletzl H, et al. Functional improvement in mouse models of familial amyotrophic lateral sclerosis by PEGylated insulin-like growth factor i treatment depends on disease severity. Amyotroph Lateral Scler. 2012;13[5]:418-29.

[55] Kranzler JH, Rosenbloom AL, Martinez V, Guevara-Aguirre J. Normal intelligence with severe insulin-like growth factor I deficiency due to growth hormone receptor deficiency: A controlled study in a genetically homogeneous population. J Clin Endocrinol Metab. 1998;83[6]:1953-8.

[56] Ashpole, Nicole M; Sanders, Jessica E; Hodges Erik L; Yan HSWE. Growth Hormone, IGF-1 and the aging brain. Exp Gerontol. 2016;68[August]:76-81.

[57] Vitale G, Pellegrino G, Vollery M, Hofland LJ. ROLE of IGF-1 system in the

modulation of longevity: Controversies and new insights from a centenarians' perspective. Front Endocrinol [Lausanne]. 2019;10[FEB]:1-11.

[58] Chaves J, Saif MW. IGF system in cancer. Anticancer Drugs. 2011;22[3]:206-12.

[59] Narasimhan SD, Yen K, Tissenbaum HA. Converging Pathways in Lifespan Regulation. Curr Biol [Internet]. 2009;19[15]:R657-66. Available from: http://dx.doi.org/10.1016/j.cub.2009.06.013

[60] Gan L, Cookson MR, Petrucelli L, La Spada AR. Converging pathways in neurodegeneration, from genetics to mechanisms [Internet]. Vol. 21, Nature Neuroscience. Nature Publishing Group; 2018 [cited 2021 Feb 4]. p. 1300-9.

[61] Mao K, Quipildor GF, Tabrizian T, Novaj A, Guan F, Walters RO, et al. Late-life targeting of the IGF-1 receptor improves healthspan and lifespan in female mice. Nat Commun [Internet]. 2018 Dec 1 [cited 2021 Feb 5];9[1]:1-12. Available from: www.nature.com/naturecommunications

[62] Longo VD, Antebi A, Bartke A, Barzilai N, Brown-Borg HM, Caruso C, et al. Interventions to slow aging in humans: Are we ready? Vol. 14, Aging Cell. Blackwell Publishing Ltd; 2015. p. 497-510.

[63] Bartke A, List EO, Kopchick JJ. The somatotropic axis and aging: Benefits of endocrine defects. Vol. 27, Growth Hormone and IGF Research. Churchill Livingstone; 2016. p. 41-5.

[64] Riikonen R. Insulin-like growth factors in the pathogenesis of neurological diseases in children [Internet]. Vol. 18, International Journal of Molecular Sciences. MDPI AG; 2017

[65] Sisley S, Gutierrez-Aguilar R, Scott M, D'Alessio D, Sandoval D, Seeley R. Neuronal GLP1R mediates liraglutide's anorectic but not glucose-lowering effect. J Clin Invest. 2014;124[6]:2456-63.

[66] Mandić M, Drinovec L, Glisic S, Veljkovic N, Nøhr J, Vrecl M. Demonstration of a direct interaction between&beta2- Adrenergic receptor and insulin receptor by BRET and bioinformatics. PLoS One. 2014;9[11].

[67] Woodall MC, Ciccarelli M, Woodall BP, Koch WJ. GRK2 – A Link Between Myocardial Contractile Function and Cardiac Metabolism. Circ Res. 2014;114[10]:1661-70.

[68] Muniyappa R, Yavuz S. Metabolic actions of angiotensin II and insulin: A microvascular endothelial balancing act. Mol Cell Endocrinol [Internet]. 2013;378[1-2]:59-69. Available from: http://dx.doi.org/10.1016/j.mce.2012.05.017

[69] Tu H, Xu C, Zhang W, Liu Q, Rondard P, Pin JP, et al. GABAB receptor activation protects neurons from apoptosis via IGF-1 receptor transactivation. J Neurosci. 2010;30[2]:749-59.

[70] Lin X, Li X, Jiang M, Chen L, Xu C, Zhang W, et al. An activity-based probe reveals dynamic protein-protein interactions mediating IGF-1R transactivation by the GABA B receptor. Biochem J. 2012;443[3]:627-34.

[71] Pyne NJ, Pyne S. Receptor tyrosine kinase-G-protein-coupled receptor signalling platforms: Out of the shadow? Trends Pharmacol Sci [Internet]. 2011;32[8]:443-50. Available from: http://dx.doi.org/10.1016/j.tips.2011.04.002

[72] Jean-Charles PY, Kaur S, Shenoy SK. G Protein-Coupled Receptor Signaling Through β-Arrestin-Dependent Mechanisms [Internet]. Vol. 70, Journal

of Cardiovascular Pharmacology. Lippincott Williams and Wilkins; 2017 [cited 2021 Feb 5]. p. 142-58.

[73] Delcourt N, Thouvenot E, Chanrion B, Galéotti N, Jouin P, Bockaert J, et al. PACAP type I receptor transactivation is essential for IGF-1 receptor signalling and antiapoptotic activity in neurons. EMBO J. 2007;26[6]:1542-51.

[74] Nash AI. Crosstalk between insulin and dopamine signaling: A basis for the metabolic effects of antipsychotic drugs. J Chem Neuroanat [Internet]. 2017;83-84:59-68. Available from: http://dx.doi.org/10.1016/j.jchemneu.2016.07.010

[75] Quan Z, Zheng D, Qing H. Regulatory roles of long non-coding rnas in the central nervous system and associated neurodegenerative diseases. Vol. 11, Frontiers in Cellular Neuroscience. Frontiers Media S.A.; 2017.

[76] Chanda K, Mukhopadhyay D. LncRNA Xist, X-chromosome Instability and Alzheimer's Disease . Curr Alzheimer Res [Internet]. 2020 Aug 8 [cited 2021 Feb 5];17[6]:499-507. Available from: https://pubmed.ncbi.nlm.nih.gov/32851944/

[77] Degirmenci U, Li J, Lim YC, Siang DTC, Lin S, Liang H, et al. Silencing an insulin-induced lncRNA, LncASIR, impairs the transcriptional response to insulin signalling in adipocytes. Sci Rep. 2019;9[1]:1-10.

[78] Chen B, Li J, Chi D, Sahnoune I, Calin S, Girnita L, et al. Non-Coding RNAs in IGF-1R Signaling Regulation : Diabetes and Cancer. 2019;

[79] Faivre E, Hölscher C. Neuroprotective effects of D-Al2GIP on Alzheimer's disease biomarkers in an APP/PS1 mouse model. Alzheimer's Res Ther. 2013;5[2].

[80] Holzenberger M, Dupont J, Ducos B, Leneuve P, Géloën A, Even PC, et al. IGF-1 receptor regulates lifespan and resistance to oxidative stress in mice. Nature. 2003 Jan 9;421[6919]:182-7.

[81] Lanni C, Masi M, Racchi M, Govoni S. Cancer and Alzheimer's disease inverse relationship: an age-associated diverging derailment of shared pathways [Internet]. Vol. 26, Molecular Psychiatry. Springer Nature; 2020 [cited 2021 Feb 5]. p. 280-95. Available from: https://doi.org/10.1038/s41380-020-0760-2

Chapter 7

Updates in Pharmacogenetics of Non-Small Cell Lung Cancer

Munindra Ruwali, Keshav Moharir, Sanjiv Singh, Punita Aggarwal and Manash K. Paul

Abstract

Though significant clinical advances have been made, lung cancer remains the most lethal, with a low 5-year survival rate. The variability in patient response towards therapy is substantial and is associated with lung cancer's genomic landscape. Pharmacogenetic studies have deciphered many clinically relevant associations between tumor genetic alterations and their influences on drug efficacy, toxicity sensitivity and overall outcomes of cancer treatment. Biomarkers are tools in the arsenal that can help in the prediction, prognosis, diagnosis and follow-up of cancer treatment. Bulk and single-cell next-generation sequencing of large patient cohorts have generated a better understanding of the genetic underpinnings of lung cancer, and opening up personalized therapeutic opportunities. Immunotherapy and personalized medicine are providing hope for lung cancer patients. This review highlights the genetic alterations and important lung cancer biomarkers. The pharmacogenetic associations, personalized immunotherapy and challenges associated with effective therapy are also discussed. Pharmacogenetics and pharmacogenomics can open up new vistas for optimized, personalized NSCLC treatment.

Keywords: Lung cancer, NSCLC, Pharmacogenetics, Biomarkers, Personalized medicine, Tyrosine kinase inhibitors, Immunotherapy, Checkpoint inhibitor, Challenges

1. Introduction

Lung cancer is the principal cause of cancer-related death worldwide and affects both smokers and non-smokers [1]. Men have the highest incidence and mortality related to lung cancer, while in women, it is third by incidence and second by mortality. With exceptions, the five-year survival rate of lung cancer patients is between 10 and 20%, the lowest among most cancer types [2]. Histologically 80–85% of lung cancers are classified as non-small cell lung cancer (NSCLC), while the remaining is small cell lung cancer (SCLC). Adenocarcinoma (LUAD; ~ 65%), squamous cell carcinoma (LUSC; ~ 30%), and large cell carcinoma (LCLC) are the major subtypes of NSCLC and originates from different types of lung cells [1, 3, 4]. While SCLC is less frequent but more aggressive as compared to LUAD and LUSC. NSCLC is mainly treated by surgery, chemotherapy, radiation, or targeted therapy but with dismal lung cancer survival outcomes. There has been extensive progress

IntechOpen

in aiming targeted drug delivery towards cancer cells; the accuracy, efficacy, and success are often limited by resistance developed by tumor cells and inter-subject variability. Low therapeutic indices, differences in health effects, and toxicity from chemotherapeutic agents are some of the drawbacks of current NSCLC treatment. This has prompted researchers to explore other cancer treatment options, keeping in mind individual patient's genetic responses and adverse drug reactions (ADR) to chemotherapeutic agents as 'pharmacogenetics' studies [5].

Pharmacogenetics is an evolving branch of pharmacology that examines the genetic variation between individuals and its correlation with their response to drugs/pharmaceuticals and other xenobiotics. In comparison, pharmacogenomics encompasses all genes in the genome that modulates drug response. The awareness of the genetic heterogeneity in oncology is of significant importance, owing to the limited therapeutic index of cancer therapies and the possibility of ADR-associated life-threatening complications. Within an individual and comparison among NSCLC patients, genomic alterations are major reasons for variations in chemotherapeutic drug response and related toxicity [6]. Studies on NSCLC genetic and molecular alterations provide new targets for treatment, help in the identification of biomarkers for early diagnosis, and helps to predict patient prognosis and progression [7]. NSCLC genetic polymorphism can act as either predictive or prognostic markers [8]. Single-nucleotide polymorphisms (SNPs) or a single nucleotide substitution can affect the expression or functionality of essential enzymes and/or targets in the metabolism and activity of anticancer drugs. Genetic polymorphism is extensively investigated as a prognostic or predictive factor in various tumor types, including NSCLC [9].

Further, pharmacogenetics also helps to prevent cancer-related mortalities by forecasting pre-symptomatic diagnosis, designing customized or tailor-made dosage regimens for individuals, and optimization of a therapeutic window of antineoplastic drugs on a personalized basis. However, pharmacogenetics is an evolving arena in cancer treatment and has obvious underlying limitations that need to be investigated. Determination of genetic variants has primarily relied on SNP, although lately, haplotypes of SNPs and non-genetic factors (like age, lifestyle, diet, profession, and intestinal microflora) are included in studies. Nonetheless, an additional challenge in pharmacogenetics for treating NSCLC deals with validation and standardization of genotyping procedures that are a major deciding factor in the personalization of cancer therapy. Many therapeutic interventions can be utilized for pharmacogenetics-associated NSCLC treatment. The examples include, but not restricted to chemotherapeutic agents (cisplatin, gemcitabine, pemetrexed, taxanes, etc.), immune checkpoint inhibitors [programmed cell death 1 (PD-1), cytotoxic T-lymphocyte protein 4 (CTLA-4)], and a combination of immunotherapy with chemotherapy [10]. This chapter throws light on the current status of pharmacogenetics-based therapeutics in NSCLC with a focus on genetic alterations by gene mutations, exploration of possible treatment modalities, challenges involved, and prospects of pharmacogenetics in treating NSCLC.

2. Gene mutation in NSCLC and Pharmacogenetics

Human Genome Project (HGP) has revealed that the genetic composition of humans is 99% similar, with only 1% variations leading to individual differences. This clarifies why individuals show a difference in response to anticancer drugs concerning drug pharmacology, toxicity, and controlling proliferation, invasion, and metastasis of tumor cells in NSCLC [11, 12]. Simultaneously, several studies have suggested a personalized medicine approach to achieving maximum efficacy and minimum toxicity of anticancer drugs using pharmacogenetics to target NSCLC [12]. Thus, NSCLC patients' categorization based on underlying genetic and molecular alterations can help in personalizing anticancer drugs and dosage regimens. Therapy tuned to individual patient's genotypic and phenotypic landscape can achieve the highest therapeutic benefits [13]. The complete knowledge of driver mutation pathways and biomarkers can explain NSCLC heterogeneity for identifying personalizing therapies. Information about driver mutation frequency and associated functional changes can help decipher actionable, personalized molecular targets. Therefore, a brief description of the critical driver genes that frequently undergo mutations-associated with lung cancer (**Figure 1**).

NSCLC is a heterogeneous disease, and recent sequencing studies have revealed the genomic landscape (**Figure 1**). Common genomic alterations in LUAD include KRAS, EGFR, HER2, MET, RET, ALK, and ROS1, while the important alteration in tumor suppressor includes TP53, KEAP1, LKB1, and NF1 (**Figure 1**) [1, 14]. Interestingly the major genomic alterations in LUSC include TP53, PIK3CA, CDKN2A, NFE2L2, KEAP1, SOX2, PTEN, CDKN2A, RB1, CCND1, NOTCH1, MLL2, and HLA-A (**Figure 1**) [1, 15] (**Figure 1**). Inhibitors of these genes are primarily used as a treatment procedure and as one of the targeted therapies. Several driver oncogenes involved in NSCLC have been identified to be targeted with prior information of molecular testing and individual patient's pharmacogenetics towards drugs employed. Examples of such targets include EGFR, ALK, KRAS, BRAF, ROS 1, PTEN, HER 2, MET, and FGFR, identified in some patient subsets of NSCLC as potential treatment targets [16].

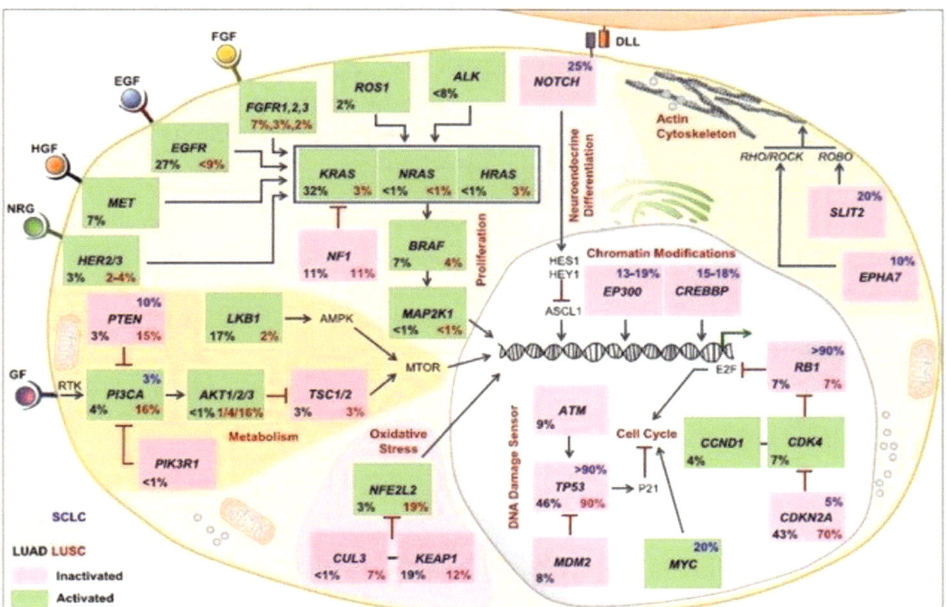

Figure 1.
Comparison of genetic changes in major oncogenic pathways in individuals with LUAD, LUSC, and SCLC and the frequencies are shown in the specific boxes. The genetic alterations data is a sum of somatic defects, homozygous deletions, focal amplifications, and major changes of gene expression. Reproduced from Salehi-Rad et al. [1].

2.1 Epidermal growth factor receptor (EGFR)

EGFR (HER1 in humans) is part of the ErbB family of receptor tyrosine kinases (RTKs). Intracellular signaling occurs when RTKs are bound extracellularly to form homo or heterodimers [17]. Clinically significant mutations occur within the tyrosine kinase domain and are associated with drug sensitivity. The genetic alteration, including mutation or amplification in EGFR, results in increased tumoral metastasis, angiogenesis, and proliferation. Multiple mutations in the EGFR tyrosine kinase domain (deletion exon 19, L858R in exon 21) are associated with NSCLC. ATP-competitive TKIs bind to EGFR and yield promising clinical outcomes. Though targeted therapy for most EGFR mutations has produced better clinical outcomes, T790M mutation inhibition in EGFR resulted in resistance to targeted therapy [18]. Three generations of TKI have been reported for personalized NSCLC precision therapy based on patient pharmacogenetics; first-generation examples being gefitinib and erlotinib, second-generation Afatinib, and Neratinib while the third generation includes osimertinib [12]. Afatinib is an irreversible TKI, which has a unique property that, unlike other TKIs it does not require CYP3A4 activity in the liver for its targeted anticancer action. Thus, NSCLC patients with pharmacogenetics of deficient or abnormal CYP3A4 activity can be treated with afatinib over other established TKIs [19].

2.2 Anaplastic lymphoma kinase (ALK) and ROS Proto-Oncogene 1 (ROS 1)

A fusion gene of anaplastic lymphoma kinase (ALK) with echinoderm microtubule-associated protein-like 4 (EML4) (EML4-ALK) is prevalent in 3–5% NSCLC patients. EML4-ALK variants act as driver mutations and modulate the JAK/STAT, PI3K/AKT, and MAPK pathways, thereby provide proliferative and survival advantages to the cancer cells. Crizotinib blocks the kinase activity of the EML4-ALK and induces cancer cell apoptosis. ALK fusion is also familiar with other genes, including HIP1, KIF5B, KLC1, DCTN1, PTPN3, STRN, and show association with NSCLC. Individuals with NSCLC having significant ALK rearrangements can be genetically identified with advanced techniques like comprehensive next-generation sequencing (NGS), immunohistochemistry, and in-situ fluorescence hybridization (FISH). In advanced NSCLC stages, ALK TKIs have confirmed the progression-free survival of patients with better prognoses. Several second-generation ALK inhibitors can help target ALK-positive NSCLC, such as alectinib, ceritinib, and AP26133 developed and are currently under evaluation in clinical trials [20]. ROS1 rearrangements are observed in 1–2% of NSCLC patients. ROS 1 is a receptor tyrosine kinase and is structurally homology to ALK protein and serves as the basis of using ALK inhibitors to target ROS1+ NSCLCs. Crizotinib and entrectinib are FDA approved and show a quick positive response by slowing cancer progression in ROS-1+ NSCLC [21].

2.3 BRAF

BRAF encodes a threonine/serine protein kinase that is an effector protein of KRAS. BRAF activates the MAPK signal transduction, which regulates cell proliferation and survival. Mutations in BRAF are about 1 to 3% in NSCLC, with a predominance of V600E (50%), G469A (39%), D594G (11%), and K601E, G469S, G596R, G466R, and T599dup [21]. Dabrafenib is a BRAF inhibitor combined with trametinib (MEK inhibitor), is FDA approved for BRAF V600E+ metastatic NSCLC. Vemurafenib, another BRAF inhibitor, showed a 42% overall response rate for BRAF V600E+ NSCLC in a basket trial.

2.4 Kristen Rat Sarcoma Viral oncogene (KRAS)

KRAS encodes a G protein and is a member of the RAS proto-oncogene family. KRAS-GTP complex activates the RAS/MAPK, PI3K/mTOR, and RalGDS-RalA/B signaling pathways and regulates cell proliferation, differentiation, and survival. Mutations in KRAS are recurrent in NSCLC (25–40%), especially LUAD. Ras gene and three forms are present H-Ras, N-Ras and K-Ras. In general, KRAS mutations have a poor prognosis. Out of KRAS mutations, G12C, G12V, G12D, and G12A are common and more frequent in male smokers. Common mutation among smokers is G12C (about 41%), while in nonsmokers, it is G12D (56%) and G12V. Though compounds are discovered that target the GDP-binding pocket (ARS-853, SML-8-73-1) but the efficacy and toxicity have been a hurdle. Currently, there is no specific developed FDA-approved anticancer agent that uniquely targets KRAS; however, MEK and PI3K/mTOR/MEK inhibitors are thought to be selective in the inhibiting downstream targets of KRAS mutant cases [22]. KRAS gain-of-function mutations serve as predictive markers for NSCLC chemotherapy, but recent studies present a geographical bias. KRAS mutations are frequent amongst westerns (30%) compared to Asian (10%) LUAD patients [23]. Moreover, the prognostic and predictive response is more efficient in LUAD than other NSCLC subtypes, and proper clinical pharmacogenetic evaluation and implementation is needed.

2.5 Receptor 2 of the human epidermal growth factor (HER2)

HER2 (ERBB2) is a proto-oncogene, encodes for tyrosine kinase receptors, and relies on heterodimerization for activation with receptors from the EFGR family. Upon activation, HER2, in turn, triggers downstream signaling like PI3K/mTOR, RAF/MEK/ERK, and the MEK/JNK pathways and regulates cell proliferation, differentiation, and migration. HER2 genetic alteration not only drives several tumors (breast and gastric cancer) but also plays a crucial role in NSCLC formation. HER2 amplification and overexpression are associated with 7–34.9% of NSCLCs and are related to poor prognosis. Activating mutations (like HER exon 20) are observed in 2–4% of NSCLCs cases, especially in LUAD [24]. The mutations in the tyrosine kinase domain are investigated as attractive therapeutic targets in NSCLC. Targeted therapy against HER2 (TKIs and antibody) is under clinical investigation, and the value of HER2 for such patient screening is gaining precedence. HER2-targeted TKIs, include afatinib, ipatinib, neratinib, and pyrotinib, while trastuzumab and T-DM1 conjugate are antibody-based [25].

2.6 REarranged during Transfection (RET)

RET proto-oncogene encodes for an RTK, localized to chromosome 10, and activates replication, cell proliferation, motility and differentiation. The GDFN family ligand (GFL) interaction with GDFN-family receptor α (GFRα) initiates RET receptor protein dimerization and formation GFL-GFRα-RET heteromeric complex. The complex formation results in RET activation and downstream signaling via RAS/RAF/MEK/ERK or PI3K/AKT1/mTOR pathways. Abnormal RET signaling may lead to cancerous growth and have a driver potential. RET Rearrangements are common in lung cancers (1–2%). RET fusions are common in NSCLC with partner genes like kinesin family member 5B (KIF5B), coiled-coil domain containing 6 (CCDC6), tripartite motif-containing 33 (TRIM33), Cut like homeobox 1 (CUX1), nuclear receptor coactivator 4 (NCOA4), and KIAA1468 [26]. Selpercatinib, a TKI that is FDA approved for use in RET+ NSCLC [27]. Other TKIs like vandetanib, cabozantinib, sorafenib and sunitinib can inhibit activated RET signaling and tumorigenic

Target gene (% mutation frequency)	Genetic alterations	Mutation effect	Drugs employed	References
EGFR [10–25]	Mutation	↑ angiogenesis, proliferation and metastasis	Gefitinib, Erlotinib, Afatinib, Neratinib, Osimertinib	[14]
EML4-ALK [2–4]	Fusion	↑ proliferation, migration and survival	Alectinib, Crizotinib, Ceritinib,	[30, 31]
ROS 1 [2, 3]	Fusion, rearrangement	↑ cell survival and resistance	Crizotinib and Foretinib	[32]
KRAS [2–5]	Mutation	↑ Chemotherapy resistance, survival and proliferation	Sorafenib, Ridaforolimus, Selumetinib + Docetaxel	[33]
MET [1, 2]	Amplification, exon 14 skipping	↑ proliferation and metastasis	Cabozantinib, Crizotinib Ornatuzumab, Tivantinib	[34]
BRAF [2, 3]	Mutation	↑ Proliferation, and survival, ↑ Resistance to EGFR inhibitors	Sorafenib, Debrafenib	[35]
RET	Fusion, rearrangement	↑ Proliferation	Carbozantinib, Ponatinib, Vandetanib	[13]
FGFR 1	Amplification	↑ chemo resistance proliferation and survival	Dovitinib Nintedanib, Ponatinib	[36]
PTEN	Deletion and mutation	↑PI3K signaling, survival and proliferation	PI3K inhibitors	[37]
PIK3CA [1–3]	Mutation	↑ Metastasis and survival	Buparlisib, inhibitors for AKT	[38]
TP53 [30–50]	Mutation	↓ apoptosis, ↑ Growth	—	[39]
DDR2	Mutation	↑ invasion and Cell migration,, proliferation and survival	Dasatinib	[40]
CDKN2A	Deletions	↑ Cell growth	—	[41]
HER2 [5–10]	Mutation	↑ Amplification	Afatinib, Dacomitinib, neratinib, Trastuzumab	[16]

Table 1.
Mutating genes associated with NSCLC, mechanism of mutation with its effects, and targeted therapy.

transformation. Activating RET mutations like M918T and acquired RET mutations (G810R, G810S, and G810C) in response to selpercatinib treatment is also reported in NSCLC [28]. Thus, RET is an interactive target and a biomarker for NSCLC.

Other actionable biomarkers in the lung include MET, PI3KCA, NTRK1, FGFR2, and DDR2 and are explained in detail elsewhere [29]. As driver mutations affect specific and exclusive cellular pathways to cause cancer, opportunities are being explored for targeted drug therapies towards various mutating genes associated with NSCLC, as mentioned in **Table 1**.

3. Genetic alterations and lung cancer treatment response

NSCLC is a widely prevalent and challenging health problem for the human race. Despite rapid advances in lung cancer treatment, it is still one of the leading causes of death worldwide. Traditional chemotherapeutic approaches failed to yield satisfactory results in terms of treatment outcome. Interestingly, the association of genetic variations with treatment outcome of some of the most commonly used chemotherapeutic drugs has opened new vistas in the domain of lung cancer treatment [12]. The relatively new area of Pharmacogenetics aims to correlate the association between genetic variations and drug effects and formulate a rational personalized drug treatment offering minimum side effects and maximum efficacy [42]. The inherited genetic variations such as single-nucleotide polymorphisms (SNPs) have been primarily studied, most commonly focusing on the candidate gene approach. These genetic changes can either lead to the altered expression or function of drug-metabolizing enzymes or their targets, thereby modulating the activity of chemotherapeutics [43].

Pemetrexed is a commonly used folate antimetabolite, a multi-targeted anti-cancer drug used in NSCLC treatment. Pemetrexed causes inhibition of critical enzymes in the folate pathway including, thymidylate synthase, dihydrofolate reductase, and glycinamide ribonucleotide formyl transferase leading to a reduction in folate depletion resulting in altered purines and pyrimidines synthesis [44]. Thymidylate synthase (TS) expression is associated with the treatment outcome, especially in nonsquamous carcinoma patients treated with pemetrexed-based chemotherapy [45]. Studies conducted on the role of polymorphisms in TS, such as polymorphic tandem repeats located in the TS enhancer region (TSER), provide conflicting results. While some studies have observed that increased expression of TS with three copies (TSER*3) of the R than with two copies (TSER*2) is associated with treatment outcome in lung cancers, other studies did not observe such an association [46]. However, the homozygous variant T677 T of methylenetetrahydrofolate reductase was associated with prolonged progression-free survival compared to the wild-type or heterozygous genotype. The observation could be due to increased TS inhibition by pemetrexed due to the polymorphic variant since methylenetetrahydrofolate reductase is an essential regulator of folate homeostasis.

The entry of pemetrexed into the cells is mediated by the reduced folate carrier (RFC). A study investigating the combined action of pemetrexed and bevacizumab suggested the role of polymorphisms in RFC exon6 and progression-free survival. A similar association was also observed with IVS7 (1478) polymorphism in glutamyl hydrolase (GGH) while GGH IVS2 (1307) CC genotype was associated with significantly longer overall survival [47]. On the contrary, no association was observed with the outcome for GGH IVS7 (1478) and IVS2 (1307) in a randomized phase II trial involving fifty four patients for treatment with pemetrexed and gemcitabine [48]. The study also reported an association of RFC-exon6-SNP with outcome following treatment with pemetrexed.

The tyrosine kinase inhibitor (TKI) family has been clinically successful as an anti-cancer strategy. An enhanced expression of EGFR leads to the activation of pathways and proto-oncogenes that can lead to lung cancer development. For the EGFR gene, most of the studies have focused on polymorphisms present in regions regulating the expression, such as those present in the 5′-flanking region and intron-1. Two important SNPs located in the transcriptional start site of the promoter region of EGFR are −191C/A and − 216G/T. The −191C/A polymorphism causes enhanced EGFR expression and activity, while the −216G/T genotype, located at the binding site for the transcription factor Sp1, increases mRNA expression. However, the A-G variant, causing substitution of an arginine with a lysine at codon 497 (R497K), leads to the reduction of EGFR activity [49]. All three polymorphisms were evaluated for association with gefitinib treatment response in advanced NSCLC patients. Out of the three polymorphisms, the −216G/T variant showed a significant association with prolonged progression-free survival, high rates of stable disease/partial response, and treatment-related side effects such as rash and diarrhea [50].

Another EGFR polymorphism present in intron one was also reported to play an important role in the treatment outcome of gefitinib for NSCLC in different ethnic groups. The dinucleotide polymorphism is associated with a variable number of CA repeats in NSCLC. Upon gefitinib-treatment, it was observed that a smaller number of CA repeats was associated with increased EGFR transcription and better survival. This was observed in both Asian and Caucasian populations. For instance, studies conducted in Chinese patients treated with gefitinib reported better responses in NSCLC patients with shorter CA repeats (less than 16 repeats) [51]. However, the results were inconsistent in Caucasian patients as no association was observed for CA repeats and clinical outcomes in patients treated with gefitinib [52]. Similar observations were also made in a study involving advanced NSCLC patients treated with erlotinib [53].

Genetic polymorphisms in Protein kinase B (AKT1), DNA repair pathway genes like ATP-binding cassette superfamily G member 2 (ABCG2) also play an essential role in determining the treatment outcome in NSCLC patients. In studies involving the Caucasian populations, lower Akt protein levels were observed associated with haplotype having two polymorphisms (SNP3 and SNP4). The same haplotype was also found associated with lower rates of apoptosis-induction by radiation in EBV-transformed lymphoblastoid. In another Caucasian study involving NSCLC patients treated with gefitinib, AKT1-SNP4 A/A genotype was associated with shorter overall survival while AKT1-rs2498804 GT and GG alleles resulted in metastases in the brain [54]. Similar observations were also made in a Korean study where it was observed that in NSCLC patients, several genetic variations in the PI3K/AKT pathway served as a useful marker in response to various chemotherapeutic drugs [55].

ABCG2 is a member of the ATP-binding cassette (ABC) transporter family and plays a crucial role in the absorption and elimination of gefitinib. ABCG2 binds gefitinib and is expressed at higher levels in the gastrointestinal tract. Polymorphisms in ABCG2 could affect the metabolism of gefitinib due to variations in expression, function, and localization of ABCG2. One such polymorphism, ABCG2 421C/A (Q141K), has been found to be associated with a decreased protein expression and associated activity of ABCG2, resulting in the accumulation of both gefitinib and erlotinib [56] though conflicting reports are also available.

Investigators have also explored the association of selected genetic variations with toxicity caused by EGFR-TKIs, such as rash and diarrhea. In a study involving 52 NSCLC patients undergoing treatment with gefitinib, different intron-1 CA repeat variants were found to be associated with varying grades of skin rash [57]. Similarly, studies have also reported the association of genetic variations in EGFR and ABCG2 with diarrhea in patients undergoing treatment with gefitinib. Examples of such variants are EGFR 191C/A and A/A, EGFR 216G/G, R497K A/A, and ABCG2 421C/A variant [50, 58]. However, another study failed to find such an association with ABCG2 421C/A, though moderate–severe diarrhea was found to be associated with ABCG2 15622C/T polymorphism and the ABCG2

(1143C/T, −15622C/T) haplotype [59]. A category of enzymes that play an essential role in the metabolism of chemotherapeutics is cytochrome P450s. Commonly used anti-cancer drugs used in the treatment of NSCLC such as gefitinib and erlotinib are metabolized by the CYP3A4, CYP3A5, and CYP1A isozymes. However, erlotinib but not gefitinib is metabolized by CYP1A2. CYPs also exhibit a large number of genetic variations, which results in different pharmacokinetics of TKIs in NSCLC patients. In cases undergoing treatment with erlotinib and having skin rash due to A/A variant of CYP3A4 resulting in lower CYP3A4 expression [60]. The same study also reported the association of CYP3A5*3 G polymorphism with grade ≥ 2 rash and diarrhea.

The ALK gene, encoding a TK receptor, gets fused with echinoderm microtubule associated protein like 4 (EML4), leading to the development of lung cancer. The fusion gene EML4-ALK encodes a fusion protein that leads to the constitutive activation of ALK kinase as a result of oligomerization of ALK in absence of the ligand. Crizotinib is a commonly used ALK-inhibitor drug that targets lung cancer caused as a result of the EML4-ALK fusion protein. It acts as a ATP-competitive inhibitor and binds to the ATP binding pocket necessary for kinase activity leading to carcinogenesis [61]. The role of ALK gene mutations in determining the treatment outcome in lung cancer patients receiving Crizotinib was brought to light when it was observed that a male patient of lung cancer developed resistance to the drug after an excellent initial response [62].

Further investigations revealed that the cause of resistance was two mutations in the ALK gene (C1156Y and L1196M). The observations were validated by an *in vitro* study in which the mutated gene, when transfected into mouse cells, resulted in reduced drug sensitivity and enhanced cellular growth when exposed to different concentrations of ALK inhibitors. In another study involving 14 ALK-positive patients, the same pattern of treatment response was observed. After promising initial response to the drug, the patients experienced tumor progression. In this study also, the reason for drug resistance was identified as mutations on the ALK gene (L1196M and G1269A) along with two more gains of copy number [63]. A study by 3D modeling into the insights of mechanisms by which the mutations alter crizotinib activity revealed that L1196M, G1202R, S1206Y and 1151insT mutants are near the crizotinib-interacting ATP-binding pocket. L1196M worked as a gatekeeper mutation as it prevents the interaction between crizotinib and the ATP-binding pocket while G1202R and S1206Y decrease affinity to crizotinib by changing the solvent-exposed region [64].

4. Antibodies and immune checkpoint inhibitors in non-small cell lung cancer

Apart from the conventional chemotherapeutic agents used for the treatment of NSCLC, immune checkpoint inhibitors (ICIs) have gained much attention in recent times. Though our immune system can target the cancer cells, yet cancer cells escape this immunosurveillance and destruction. The main hallmark of anti-tumor immune response is T cell-mediated identification of tumor-specific antigens. Tumor cell often activates immune checkpoints to effect an immune escape. Programmed cell death protein 1 (PD-1/CD279) and cytotoxic T-lymphocyte protein 4 (CTLA4) are the best-studied checkpoint inhibitors. Programmed cell death ligand-1 (PD-L1) expression, especially by tumor cells, can inhibit the response of PD-1 expressing effector T cells and induce T cell exhaustion. Treatment using anti-PD-1 or anti-PD-L1 antibody causes checkpoint blockade and thereby releases the inhibitory brake on anti-tumor effector T cell function [65, 66]. The approved monoclonal antibodies for targeting PD-1 are nivolumab and pembrolizumab while the anti-PDL1 antibodies are atezolizumab and durvalumab for lung cancer treatment [67]. The effects of pembrolizumab may be influenced by two possibilities: change in its binding site on the receptor or genetic changes that may reduce the immune system's capability to target cancer cells. A study conducted on cases showing resistance against pembrolizumab did reveal mutations that inactivated Janus kinase1 (JAK1), Janus kinase2 (JAK2), and β2 microglobulin (B2M). The data indicated that the immunological pathways were affected by the mutations [68].

CTLA-4, also known as CD152, is a receptor expressed on the surface of lymphocytes and fibroblasts. This receptor on the surface of T lymphocytes competes with CD28 (co-stimulatory receptor) to bind to the B7 ligands CD80 and CD86, expressed on the surface of antigen-presenting cells. Since the CTLA4 receptor has a higher affinity for binding to the B7 ligands, it inhibits the binding of CD28, which leads to the decreased production of the cytokine IL-2 and ultimately prevents the activity of the Cancer-Immunity Cycle (CIC) [69]. Thus, inhibition of CTLA4 checkpoint can lead to the suppression of binding between CTLA4 receptor and ligand B7. This will boost the clearance of cancer cells by activating the innate and adaptive components of the immune system. US FDA has already approved ipilimumab and tremelimumab as immune checkpoint inhibitors targeting the CTLA4 for patients with metastatic melanoma. Moreover, studies are going on with immune checkpoint inhibitors targeting the CTLA4 for NSCLC and may deliver promising results [70].

The field of immunotherapy has shown significant advancements in the treatment of several cancers, including NSCLC. However, the success is also accompanied by serious challenges, particularly in NSCLC. Some NSCLC patients show primary resistance and are unresponsive to ICIs, while others develop secondary resistance during/after the treatment. Moreover, a unique spectrum of immune-related adverse events (IRAEs) also limits the use of ICIs. The mechanism governing both the primary and secondary resistance needs further investigation. Immunopharmacogenomics can explain these resistance mechanisms. The current phase III studies of PD-1 and PD-L1 inhibitors, either alone or in combination with conventional approaches in different stages of NSCLC, will serve to improve the treatment outcome significantly [1]. However, there are still many challenges ahead though immunotherapy with checkpoint inhibitor has already raised new hopes of novel treatment modality with better and more effective treatment outcomes for NSCLC patients.

5. Challenges in pharmacogenetics in lung cancer

Lung cancer is one of the leading causes of cancer-related death worldwide, with a 5-year survival rate of approximately 15%, suggesting a comprehensive genomic alteration map may help. The lack of an early diagnosis and inefficiency in conventional therapies causes poor prognosis and lung cancer patients' overall survival. Moreover, pharmacogenetic trials ended in conflicting and inconclusive data because of non-standardized methodologies, sample heterogeneity, clinical sample processing techniques, and the inadequate number of enrolled individuals. Clinical sample preparation protocols are varied and challenging to follow in a clinical setting. Collection of needle biopsy of lung tumor is a challenge in itself. The tumor cores are usually retained as Formalin-Fixed Paraffin-Embedded (FFPE) tissue specimens. Defining the normal tissue needs more attention than we think. Recent findings suggest that normal-looking tissue adjacent to the tumor may be existing in an intermediate state. Considering tumor variability, it is unclear whether core biopsies are indicative of the oligoclonal nature of NSCLC? Data generated from specific experiments suggest histological markers can vary significantly and therefore contributing to sequence data heterogeneity within and amongst various studies. Another aspect related to biomarkers is robustness, sensitivity, and false-positive assessment of the molecular diagnostic, especially regarding immune checkpoint therapy.

Lack of pharmacogenetics biomarkers is another challenge for NSCLC pharmacogenetics. Biomarkers are significant in drug development and are used to measure the investigational drug effects on people. Cancer biomarkers are essential for diagnosis, risk assessment, the staging of cancer, screening, patient stratification, prognosis, and predict the impact of the therapy [71]. The selection of cytostatic drugs is based on the estimated responsiveness as per the predictive molecular biomarkers. In NSCLC, the predictive biomarkers that are providing for targeted therapy include EGFR and ALK. As an example, FDA-approved drugs like afatinib are associated with biomarker EGFR, and ceritinib is related to the biomarker ALK. Other essential genomic alterations in key genes like KRAS, ROS1, MET, NTRK1, FGFR, BRAF, PI3KCA, RET, PTEN, and DDR2 provide valuable information (**Figure 2**). The REMARK (Reporting Recommendations for Tumor Marker Prognostic Studies) guidelines provides criterion and suggestions for designing prognostic and tumor biomarker studies [72]. Several NSCLC studies still do not follow and comply with the standardization protocols of REMARK, thus obfuscating the clinical use scenario of biomarkers. Many trials do not include biomarker analysis as a criterion for including patients, especially in NSCLC, and serves as a significant challenge by creating selection bias. Tumor prognostic biomarker staining (for TUBB3) and scoring was done in a fraction of NSCLC in the N + IFCT-0002 trial [73].

Immune checkpoint therapy relies on monoclonal antibodies and may mediate a variety of adverse hypersensitivities, including anaphylaxis (type I), cytotoxic (type II), immune (type III), and T cell-mediated (type IV) reactions [74]. The Discovery of predictive biomarkers for immune-associated adverse reactions are essential pharmacogenetic needs for personalized cancer therapy. Genetic polymorphism, especially in the genes associated with antibody recognition, presentation, and immune response, may affect the efficacy. The role of polymorphism

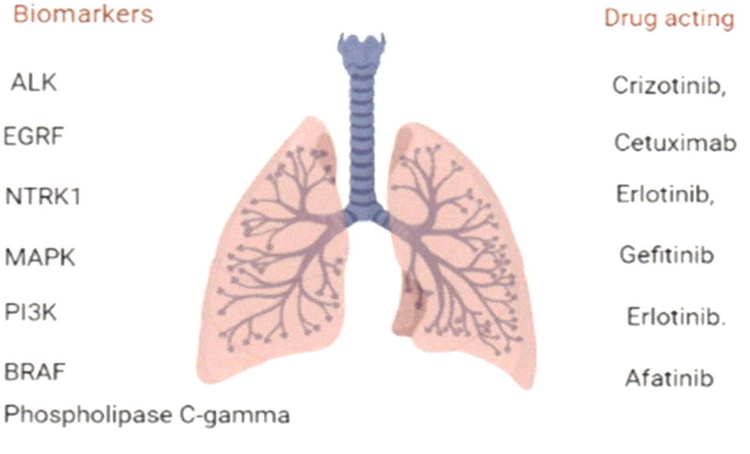

Figure 2.
Representation of biomarkers and targeting drug acting on the same.

concerning the metabolism of therapeutic antibodies can alter antibody half-life and therapeutic response. Genotypic variation in the PD-L1 (rs4143815 C/C and C/G genotype in comparison to G/G phenotype) show higher progression-free survival upon treatment with nivolumab in NSCLC [75]. A study conducted by Rizvi et al. showed a correlation of pembrolizumab efficacy with an increased nonsynonymous somatic mutational burden. A higher mutational burden was associated with an expanded neo-antigen repertoire and effective T cell-specific response [76, 77]. The Discovery of personalized biomarkers for risk assessment, detection, diagnostic, prognostic, and monitoring can be crucial in tailored NSCLC therapy. Pharmacogenetic studies correlating genetic alterations regarding immunotherapy are yet to be correctly established.

6. Future direction and conclusion

In this modern world of fast-growing medicine and research, treatment is not just about curing an aliment but also providing a better standard of life and living. With new social standards, smoking habits, and environmental pollution, NSCLC diagnoses are projected at approximately 116,660 women and 119,100 men in 2021. To treat lung cancer, it is essential to identify the disease at the earliest. The Discovery of NSCLC biomarkers can help identify disease susceptibility and aid in disease screening, diagnosis, prognosis, prediction of response, and monitoring disease recurrence. Recent advances in novel detection techniques like high throughput omics technology, multiplexed immunofluorescence microscopy, bioluminescence resonance energy transfer (BRET), CRISPR-based biosensors, surface-enhanced Raman spectroscopy have generated hope for better treatment. Bulk and single-cell next-generation sequencing (NGS), circulating cell-free DNA (cfDNA), single-cell proteomics can help in biomarker discovery and push modern pharmacogenetics and personalized medicine. Discovery strategies including hotspot panels (frequently observed gene mutations), Actionable gene panels (targeted gene exons), disease-focused panel (genes involved in a disease), comprehensive panels (correlative genes), and validated panels (tested genes) NGS applications can reduce biomarker discovery time. Machine learning-based data analyses platforms and algorithms may help undertake candidate polymorphism search; candidate pathway searches better predict correlations between gene alterations and therapeutic response.

Exploring new molecular signature-based personalized medicine can open up future potential healthcare environments. Considering the massive expansion in NGS-based NSCLC molecular data generation, integrating pharmacogenetics and genomic knowledge with the potential of theranostics can lead to effective therapy. Theranostics, the fusion of therapeutics and diagnostics, using a nanotechnology-based delivery platform can pave the way to precision and personalized medicine [78]. Nanotechnology is a quickly evolving biomedical research area and has been used to address several biological issues, including therapeutics and diagnostics [79]. Nanoscale-based delivery platforms like liposomes, polymeric nanoparticles, metal nanoparticles, and bio-nano particles can be efficiently used for theranostic applications for targeting cancer. Nanoparticle offers a benefit over standard medicinal therapies regarding biocompatibility, enhanced permeability retention, higher drug loading, targeting precision, a significant degree of versatility, and real-time monitoring of the disease [80]. Nanoparticle-based nanotheranostics can provide multifunctional benefits including, imaging, prognostic, diagnostics, and monitoring therapeutic outcome in NSCLC patients. Mukherjee et al. presented a detailed analysis of lung cancer theranostics [4].

Liquid biopsy and microfluidic technology can help in early disease detection. NGS has already helped identify new cancer-driving mutations, and this has encouraged scientists for drug repurposing. Scientists are deciphering synthetic lethality interactions, where two or more gene simultaneous alteration in the presence of a therapeutic may lead to lethality. Efficacy of immune checkpoint therapies is associated with genotypic variance, and immune-based biomarkers may provide a clear understanding of immunepharmacogenetics. Big data analyses of the growing pharmacogenetic or pharmacogenomic dataset can soon lead us to personalized NSCLC therapeutics.

Acknowledgements

Dr. Manash K. Paul acknowledges Professors, Steven Dubinett, Brigitte Gomperts and Volker Hartenstein for providing continuous support and mentoring.

Conflicts of interest

The authors declare no conflict of interest. The authors have no other pertinent affiliations or financial connection with any organization or entity with a financial interest in or financial conflict with the subject matter or materials discussed in the manuscript apart from those disclosed.

Author contributions

Conceptualization - MKP; writing original draft preparation - MR, KM, SS, PA, MKP; Review and editing - MKP.

Author details

Munindra Ruwali[1†], Keshav Moharir[2†], Sanjiv Singh[3†], Punita Aggarwal[3] and Manash K. Paul[4*]

1 Amity Institute of Biotechnology, Amity University Haryana, Gurgaon (Manesar), Haryana, India

2 Gurunanak College of Pharmacy, Nagpur, India

3 National Institute of Pharmaceutical Education and Research, Export Promotion Industrial Park (EPIP), Hajipur, Bihar, India

4 Department of Pulmonary and Critical Care Medicine, David Geffen School of Medicine, University of California Los Angeles (UCLA), Los Angeles, CA, USA

*Address all correspondence to: paul_cancerbiotech@yahoo.co.in and manashp@ucla.edu

† Equal contribution.

References

[1] Salehi-Rad R, Li R, Paul MK, Dubinett SM, Liu B. The Biology of Lung Cancer. Clinics in Chest Medicine. 2020;41(1):25-38.

[2] Sung H, Ferlay J, Siegel RL, Laversanne M, Soerjomataram I, Jemal A, et al. Global cancer statistics 2020: GLOBOCAN estimates of incidence and mortality worldwide for 36 cancers in 185 countries. CA: A Cancer Journal for Clinicians. 2021.

[3] Lai Y-H, Chen W-N, Hsu T-C, Lin C, Tsao Y, Wu S. Overall survival prediction of non-small cell lung cancer by integrating microarray and clinical data with deep learning. Scientific Reports. 2020;10(1).

[4] Mukherjee A, Paul M, Mukherjee S. Recent Progress in the Theranostics Application of Nanomedicine in Lung Cancer. Cancers. 2019;11(5).

[5] Miteva-Marcheva NN, Ivanov HY, Dimitrov DK, Stoyanova VK. Application of pharmacogenetics in oncology. Biomarker Research. 2020;8(1).

[6] D'Antonio C, Milano A, Righini R, Onesti CE, Bassanelli M, Falcone R, et al. Pharmacogenomics in lung cancer chemotherapy: a review of what the oncologist should know. Anticancer Res. 2014;34(10):5241-50.

[7] Carper MB, Claudio PP. Clinical potential of gene mutations in lung cancer. Clinical and Translational Medicine. 2015;4(1).

[8] Santarpia M, Rolfo C, Peters GJ, Leon LG, Giovannetti E. On the pharmacogenetics of non-small cell lung cancer treatment. Expert Opin Drug Metab Toxicol. 2016;12(3):307-17.

[9] Hildebrandt MA, Gu J, Wu X. Pharmacogenomics of platinum-based chemotherapy in NSCLC. Expert Opin Drug Metab Toxicol. 2009;5(7):745-55.

[10] Onoi K, Chihara Y, Uchino J, Shimamoto T, Morimoto Y, Iwasaku M, et al. Immune Checkpoint Inhibitors for Lung Cancer Treatment: A Review. Journal of Clinical Medicine. 2020;9(5).

[11] Gogtay NJ, Thatte UM, Ravi R, Bose D. Personalizing medicine with pharmacogenetics and pharmacogenomics. Clinical Molecular Medicine2020. p. 521-34.

[12] Jiang W, Cai G, Hu PC, Wang Y. Personalized medicine in non-small cell lung cancer: a review from a pharmacogenomics perspective. Acta Pharmaceutica Sinica B. 2018;8(4):530-8.

[13] Bronte G, Ulivi P, Verlicchi A, Cravero P, Delmonte A, Crinò L. Targeting RET-rearranged non-small-cell lung cancer: future prospects. Lung Cancer: Targets and Therapy. 2019;Volume 10:27-36.

[14] Comprehensive molecular profiling of lung adenocarcinoma. Nature. 2014;511(7511):543-50.

[15] Comprehensive genomic characterization of squamous cell lung cancers. Nature. 2012;489(7417):519-25.

[16] Torigoe H, Shien K, Takeda T, Yoshioka T, Namba K, Sato H, et al. Therapeutic strategies for afatinib-resistant lung cancer harboring HER2 alterations. Cancer Science. 2018;109(5):1493-502.

[17] Paul MK, Mukhopadhyay AK. Tyrosine kinase – Role and significance in Cancer. International Journal of Medical Sciences. 2004:101-15.

[18] Tartarone A, Lazzari C, Lerose R, Conteduca V, Improta G, Zupa A, et al.

Mechanisms of resistance to EGFR tyrosine kinase inhibitors gefitinib/erlotinib and to ALK inhibitor crizotinib. Lung Cancer. 2013;81(3):328-36.

[19] Wu Y-L, Zhou C, Hu C-P, Feng J, Lu S, Huang Y, et al. Afatinib versus cisplatin plus gemcitabine for first-line treatment of Asian patients with advanced non-small-cell lung cancer harbouring EGFR mutations (LUX-Lung 6): an open-label, randomised phase 3 trial. The Lancet Oncology. 2014;15(2):213-22.

[20] Sullivan I, Planchard D. ALK inhibitors in non-small cell lung cancer: the latest evidence and developments. Ther Adv Med Oncol. 2016;8(1):32-47.

[21] El-Telbany A, Ma PC. Cancer Genes in Lung Cancer: Racial Disparities: Are There Any? Genes & Cancer. 2012;3(7-8):467-80.

[22] Cicek Y, Kosar P, Öztürk Ö. Molecular genetics of lung cancer. Eurasian Journal of Pulmonology. 2018;20(3).

[23] Ghimessy A, Radeczky P, Laszlo V, Hegedus B, Renyi-Vamos F, Fillinger J, et al. Current therapy of KRAS-mutant lung cancer. Cancer and Metastasis Reviews. 2020;39(4):1159-77.

[24] Villalobos P, Wistuba II. Lung Cancer Biomarkers. Hematology/Oncology Clinics of North America. 2017;31(1):13-29.

[25] Ekman S. HER2: defining a Neu target in non-small-cell lung cancer. Annals of Oncology. 2019;30(3):353-5.

[26] Loh Z, Mitchell P, John T, Arulananda S. RET-rearranged non-small-cell lung cancer and therapeutic implications. Internal Medicine Journal. 2019;49(12):1541-5.

[27] Drilon A, Oxnard GR, Tan DSW, Loong HHF, Johnson M, Gainor J, et al. Efficacy of Selpercatinib in RET Fusion–Positive Non–Small-Cell Lung Cancer. New England Journal of Medicine. 2020;383(9):813-24.

[28] Solomon BJ, Tan L, Lin JJ, Wong SQ, Hollizeck S, Ebata K, et al. RET Solvent Front Mutations Mediate Acquired Resistance to Selective RET Inhibition in RET-Driven Malignancies. Journal of Thoracic Oncology. 2020;15(4):541-9.

[29] Cagle PT, Raparia K, Portier BP. Emerging Biomarkers in Personalized Therapy of Lung Cancer. Lung Cancer and Personalized Medicine: Novel Therapies and Clinical Management. Advances in Experimental Medicine and Biology2016. p. 25-36.

[30] Lu S, Lu C, Xiao Y, Zhu W, He Q, Xie B, et al. Comparison of EML4-ALK fusion gene positive rate in different detection methods and samples of non-small cell lung cancer. Journal of Cancer. 2020;11(6):1525-31.

[31] Wang F, Qin J, Xie F, Wu Q, Lu H. Transformation of EML4-ALK fusion-positive adenocarcinoma into squamous cell carcinoma in association with acquired resistance to crizotinib. Lung Cancer. 2020;140:118-20.

[32] Califano R, Abidin A, Tariq N-u-A, Economopoulou P, Metro G, Mountzios G. Beyond EGFR and ALK inhibition: Unravelling and exploiting novel genetic alterations in advanced non small-cell lung cancer. Cancer Treatment Reviews. 2015;41(5):401-11.

[33] Salgia R, Pharaon R, Mambetsariev I, Nam A, Sattler M. The improbable targeted therapy: KRAS as an emerging target in non-small cell lung cancer (NSCLC). Cell Reports Medicine. 2021;2(1).

[34] Wang Q, Yang S, Wang K, Sun S-Y. MET inhibitors for targeted therapy of

EGFR TKI-resistant lung cancer. Journal of Hematology & Oncology. 2019;12(1).

[35] Bustamante JG, Otterson GA. Agents to treat BRAF-mutant lung cancer. Drugs in Context. 2019;8:1-5.

[36] Giacomini A, Taranto S, Rezzola S, Matarazzo S, Grillo E, Bugatti M, et al. Inhibition of the FGF/FGFR System Induces Apoptosis in Lung Cancer Cells via c-Myc Downregulation and Oxidative Stress. International Journal of Molecular Sciences. 2020;21(24).

[37] Liu L, Huang L, He J, Cai S, Weng Y, Huang S, et al. PTEN inhibits non-small cell lung cancer cell growth by promoting G0/G1 arrest and cell apoptosis. Oncology Letters. 2018.

[38] Yang J, Nie J, Ma X, Wei Y, Peng Y, Wei X. Targeting PI3K in cancer: mechanisms and advances in clinical trials. Molecular Cancer. 2019;18(1).

[39] Duffy MJ, Synnott NC, Crown J. Mutant p53 as a target for cancer treatment. European Journal of Cancer. 2017;83:258-65.

[40] Osei E, Lumini J, Gunasekara D, Osei B, Asare A, Laflamme R. A review of predictive, prognostic and diagnostic biomarkers for non-small-cell lung cancer: towards personalised and targeted cancer therapy. Journal of Radiotherapy in Practice. 2019;19(4):370-84.

[41] Liu W, Zhuang C, Huang T, Yang S, Zhang M, Lin B, et al. Loss of CDKN2A at chromosome 9 has a poor clinical prognosis and promotes lung cancer progression. Molecular Genetics & Genomic Medicine. 2020;8(12).

[42] Ruwali M. Pharmacogenetics and Cancer Treatment: Progress and Prospects. Molecular Medicine2019.

[43] Giovannetti E, Toffalorio F, De Pas T, Peters GJ. Pharmacogenetics of conventional chemotherapy in non-small-cell lung cancer: a changing landscape? Pharmacogenomics. 2012;13(9):1073-86.

[44] Galvani E, Peters GJ, Giovannetti E. Thymidylate synthase inhibitors for non-small cell lung cancer. Expert Opinion on Investigational Drugs. 2011;20(10):1343-56.

[45] Sun J-M, Han J, Ahn JS, Park K, Ahn M-J. Significance of Thymidylate Synthase and Thyroid Transcription Factor 1 Expression in Patients with Nonsquamous Non-small Cell Lung Cancer Treated with Pemetrexed-Based Chemotherapy. Journal of Thoracic Oncology. 2011;6(8):1392-9.

[46] Tiseo M, Giovannetti E, Tibaldi C, Camerini A, Di Costanzo F, Barbieri F, et al. Pharmacogenetic study of patients with advanced non-small cell lung cancer (NSCLC) treated with second-line pemetrexed or pemetrexed–carboplatin. Lung Cancer. 2012;78(1):92-9.

[47] Adjei AA, Mandrekar SJ, Dy GK, Molina JR, Adjei AA, Gandara DR, et al. Phase II Trial of Pemetrexed Plus Bevacizumab for Second-Line Therapy of Patients With Advanced Non–Small-Cell Lung Cancer: NCCTG and SWOG Study N0426. Journal of Clinical Oncology. 2010;28(4):614-9.

[48] Adjei AA, Salavaggione OE, Mandrekar SJ, Dy GK, Ziegler KLA, Endo C, et al. Correlation Between Polymorphisms of the Reduced Folate Carrier Gene (SLC19A1) and Survival After Pemetrexed-Based Therapy in Non-small Cell Lung Cancer: A North Central Cancer Treatment Group-Based Exploratory Study. Journal of Thoracic Oncology. 2010;5(9):1346-53.

[49] Heist RS, Christiani D. EGFR-targeted therapies in lung cancer: predictors of response and toxicity. Pharmacogenomics. 2009;10(1):59-68.

[50] Liu G, Gurubhagavatula S, Zhou W, Wang Z, Yeap BY, Asomaning K, et al. Epidermal growth factor receptor polymorphisms and clinical outcomes in non-small-cell lung cancer patients treated with gefitinib. The Pharmacogenomics Journal. 2007;8(2):129-38.

[51] Nie Q, Wang Z, Zhang G-c, An S-j, Lin J-y, Guo A-l, et al. The epidermal growth factor receptor intron1 (CA) n microsatellite polymorphism is a potential predictor of treatment outcome in patients with advanced lung cancer treated with Gefitinib. European Journal of Pharmacology. 2007;570(1-3):175-81.

[52] Gregorc V, Hidalgo M, Spreafico A, Cusatis G, Ludovini V, Ingersoll RG, et al. Germline Polymorphisms in EGFR and Survival in Patients With Lung Cancer Receiving Gefitinib. Clinical Pharmacology & Therapeutics. 2007;83(3):477-84.

[53] Brugger W, Triller N, Blasinska-Morawiec M, Curescu S, Sakalauskas R, Manikhas GM, et al. Prospective Molecular Marker Analyses of EGFR and KRAS From a Randomized, Placebo-Controlled Study of Erlotinib Maintenance Therapy in Advanced Non–Small-Cell Lung Cancer. Journal of Clinical Oncology. 2011;29(31):4113-20.

[54] Avan A, Maftouh M, Avan A, Tibaldi C, Zucali PA, Giovannetti E. SNPs in PI3K-PTEN-mTOR and Brain Metastases in NSCLC—Letter. Clinical Cancer Research. 2014;20(13):3623-4.

[55] Kim MJ, Kang H-G, Lee SY, Jeon H-S, Lee W-K, Park JY, et al. AKT1 polymorphisms and survival of early stage non-small cell lung cancer. Journal of Surgical Oncology. 2012;105(2):167-74.

[56] Li J, Cusatis G, Brahmer J, Sparreboom A, Robey RW, Bates SE, et al. Association of variant ABCG2 and the pharmacokinetics of epidermal growth factor receptor tyrosine kinase inhibitors in cancer patients. Cancer Biology & Therapy. 2014;6(3):432-8.

[57] Huang C-L, Yang C-H, Yeh K-H, Hu F-C, Chen K-Y, Shih J-Y, et al. EGFR intron 1 dinucleotide repeat polymorphism is associated with the occurrence of skin rash with gefitinib treatment. Lung Cancer. 2009;64(3):346-51.

[58] Morales-Espinosa D, García-Román S, Karachaliou N, Rosell R. Pharmacogenomics in the treatment of lung cancer: an update. Pharmacogenomics. 2015;16(15):1751-60.

[59] Lemos C, Giovannetti E, Zucali PA, Assaraf YG, Scheffer GL, van der Straaten T, et al. Impact ofABCG2polymorphisms on the clinical outcome and toxicity of gefitinib in non-small-cell lung cancer patients. Pharmacogenomics. 2011;12(2):159-70.

[60] Rudin CM, Liu W, Desai A, Karrison T, Jiang X, Janisch L, et al. Pharmacogenomic and Pharmacokinetic Determinants of Erlotinib Toxicity. Journal of Clinical Oncology. 2008;26(7):1119-27.

[61] Gridelli C, Peters S, Sgambato A, Casaluce F, Adjei AA, Ciardiello F. ALK inhibitors in the treatment of advanced NSCLC. Cancer Treatment Reviews. 2014;40(2):300-6.

[62] Choi YL, Soda M, Yamashita Y, Ueno T, Takashima J, Nakajima T, et al. EML4-ALK Mutations in Lung Cancer That Confer Resistance to ALK Inhibitors. New England Journal of Medicine. 2010;363(18):1734-9.

[63] Doebele RC, Pilling AB, Aisner DL, Kutateladze TG, Le AT, Weickhardt AJ, et al. Mechanisms of Resistance to Crizotinib in Patients with ALK Gene

Rearranged Non–Small Cell Lung Cancer. Clinical Cancer Research. 2012;18(5):1472-82.

[64] Katayama R, Shaw AT, Khan TM, Mino-Kenudson M, Solomon BJ, Halmos B, et al. Mechanisms of Acquired Crizotinib Resistance in ALK-Rearranged Lung Cancers. Science Translational Medicine. 2012;4(120):120ra17-ra17.

[65] Xia L, Liu Y, Wang Y. PD-1/PD-L1 Blockade Therapy in Advanced Non-Small-Cell Lung Cancer: Current Status and Future Directions. Oncologist. 2019;24(Suppl 1):S31-s41.

[66] Lee MH, Yanagawa J, Tran L, Walser TC, Bisht B, Fung E, et al. FRA1 contributes to MEK-ERK pathway-dependent PD-L1 upregulation by KRAS mutation in premalignant human bronchial epithelial cells. Am J Transl Res. 2020;12(2):409-27.

[67] Herbst RS, Baas P, Kim D-W, Felip E, Pérez-Gracia JL, Han J-Y, et al. Pembrolizumab versus docetaxel for previously treated, PD-L1-positive, advanced non-small-cell lung cancer (KEYNOTE-010): a randomised controlled trial. The Lancet. 2016;387(10027):1540-50.

[68] Zaretsky JM, Garcia-Diaz A, Shin DS, Escuin-Ordinas H, Hugo W, Hu-Lieskovan S, et al. Mutations Associated with Acquired Resistance to PD-1 Blockade in Melanoma. New England Journal of Medicine. 2016;375(9):819-29.

[69] Qureshi OS, Zheng Y, Nakamura K, Attridge K, Manzotti C, Schmidt EM, et al. Trans-Endocytosis of CD80 and CD86: A Molecular Basis for the Cell-Extrinsic Function of CTLA-4. Science. 2011;332(6029):600-3.

[70] Hellmann MD, Ciuleanu T-E, Pluzanski A, Lee JS, Otterson GA, Audigier-Valette C, et al. Nivolumab plus Ipilimumab in Lung Cancer with a High Tumor Mutational Burden. New England Journal of Medicine. 2018;378(22):2093-104.

[71] Diamandis EP. Cancer biomarkers: can we turn recent failures into success? J Natl Cancer Inst. 2010;102(19):1462-7.

[72] Sauerbrei W, Taube SE, McShane LM, Cavenagh MM, Altman DG. Reporting Recommendations for Tumor Marker Prognostic Studies (REMARK): An Abridged Explanation and Elaboration. JNCI: Journal of the National Cancer Institute. 2018;110(8):803-11.

[73] Levallet G, Bergot E, Antoine M, Creveuil C, Santos AO, Beau-Faller M, et al. High TUBB3 Expression, an Independent Prognostic Marker in Patients with Early Non–Small Cell Lung Cancer Treated by Preoperative Chemotherapy, Is Regulated by K-Ras Signaling Pathway. Molecular Cancer Therapeutics. 2012;11(5):1203-13.

[74] Shek D, Read SA, Ahlenstiel G, Piatkov I. Pharmacogenetics of anticancer monoclonal antibodies. Cancer Drug Resistance. 2019.

[75] Nomizo T, Ozasa H, Tsuji T, Funazo T, Yasuda Y, Yoshida H, et al. Clinical Impact of Single Nucleotide Polymorphism in PD-L1 on Response to Nivolumab for Advanced Non-Small-Cell Lung Cancer Patients. Scientific Reports. 2017;7(1).

[76] Rizvi NA, Hellmann MD, Snyder A, Kvistborg P, Makarov V, Havel JJ, et al. Mutational landscape determines sensitivity to PD-1 blockade in non–small cell lung cancer. Science. 2015;348(6230):124-8.

[77] Salehi-Rad R, Li R, Tran LM, Lim RJ, Abascal J, Momcilovic M, et al. Novel Kras-mutant murine models of non-small cell lung cancer possessing co-occurring oncogenic mutations and

increased tumor mutational burden. Cancer Immunology, Immunotherapy. 2021.

[78] Madamsetty VS, Paul MK, Mukherjee A, Mukherjee S. Functionalization of Nanomaterials and Their Application in Melanoma Cancer Theranostics. ACS Biomaterials Science & Engineering. 2019;6(1):167-81.

[79] Mukherjee S, Madamsetty VS, Bhattacharya D, Roy Chowdhury S, Paul MK, Mukherjee A. Recent Advancements of Nanomedicine in Neurodegenerative Disorders Theranostics. Advanced Functional Materials. 2020;30(35).

[80] Mukherjee A, Madamsetty VS, Paul MK, Mukherjee S. Recent Advancements of Nanomedicine towards Antiangiogenic Therapy in Cancer. International Journal of Molecular Sciences. 2020;21(2).

Chapter 8

Pharmacogenomics of "Core" Essential Medicines

Molungoa Sello

Abstract

Pharmacogenomics uses information about a person's genetic makeup to choose the drugs dosage regimens that are likely to work best for that particular person. The genomic research has changed the "one size fits all" approach and opened the door to more personalized approaches that consider individual genetic makeup tend to enhance the efficacy and safety of drugs; thus saving time and money. Patient DNA influences multiple steps in which the drugs interact with the body and where will the drug act in the body. Genetic makeup-based prescription, design, and implementation of therapy do not only improve the outcome of treatments, but also reduce the risk of toxicity and other adverse events. The aim of the chapter is to explore the documented pharmacogenomics of essential as per pharmacogenomic biomarkers in drug labeling; and suggest efficacy and safety modifications. Polymorphism of drug metabolizing enzymes has the greatest effect on inter individual variability of drug response; affecting the response of individuals to drugs used in the treatment of diseases. Also, genetic deficiency of some enzymes limits effectiveness of drugs in treating concerned diseases. Gene testing prior to initiating concerned treatment is the best clinical practice that to enhance the efficacy and safety of drugs.

Keywords: Pharmacogenomics, 21st WHO essential medicines "core" list, genetic testing

1. Introduction

The National Institute of General Medical Sciences define pharmacogenomics (or pharmacogenetics) as is a field of research that studies how a person's genes affect how he or she responds to medications [1]. The Centers for Disease Control (CDC) have regarded pharmacogenomics as an important example of precision medicine whereby medical treatment is tailored for each patient; based on individual genetic makeup [2]. The National Human Genome Research Institute further contended that Pharmacogenomics uses information about a person's genetic makeup (or genome) to choose the drugs and dosages that are likely to work best for that particular person. The field is an amalgam of two fields; namely pharmacology (the science of how drugs work) and genomics (the science of the human genome) [3].

The long term goal of pharmacogenomics is to help doctors select the drugs and dosage regimens best suited for each person. This is done in order to eliminate the ancient perspective that drugs have been developed with the idea that each drug works pretty much the same in everybody. But genomic research has changed that "one size fits all" approach and opened the door to more personalized approaches to using and developing drugs [3]. The approaches that consider individual genetic makeup tend to enhance the efficacy and safety of drugs; thus saving time and money.

The World Health Organization (WHO) defines essential medicines as those medicines that satisfy the priority health care needs of the population and are selected with due regard to evidence on efficacy and safety, and comparative cost-effectiveness. Essential medicines are intended to be available within the context of a well-functioning healthcare system at all times in adequate quantities, in the appropriate dosage forms, with assured quality and adequate information, and at a cost the individual and the community can afford [4]. Since 1977, WHO developed a model Essential Medicines List (EML) that could be adapted by member states in order to keep essential medicines up to date in a healthcare system. The current version of the list is the 21st WHO EML updated in June 2019 [5].

With the background given above about pharmacogenomics and essential medicines, the aim of the chapter is to explore the documented pharmacogenomics of essential medicines "**core list**" of 21st WHO EML as per United States Food and Drug Administration (USFDA) Table of Pharmacogenomic Biomarkers in Drug Labeling updated in June 2020 [6]; and suggest therapeutic modifications that can be done in order to enhance efficacy and safety of essential medicines.

1.1 How pharmacogenomics work

Patient DNA influences multiple steps in which the drugs interact with the body and where will the drug act in the body.

1.1.1 Drug receptors

In order to interact with the body, most drugs associate with cellular molecules called receptors. The receptor is the component of a cell or organism that interacts with a drug and initiates the chain of events leading to the drug's observed effects [7]. The patient genetic makeup (DNA) determines the type of receptors to have and their quantities, which can affect the response to the drug. As illustrated in **Figure 1** below, some individuals might need a higher or lower amount of the drug than most people or a different drug.

A living example of this kind of a scenario is the case of Trastuzumab emtansine (T-DM1) and breast cancer tumors with or without human epidermal growth factor

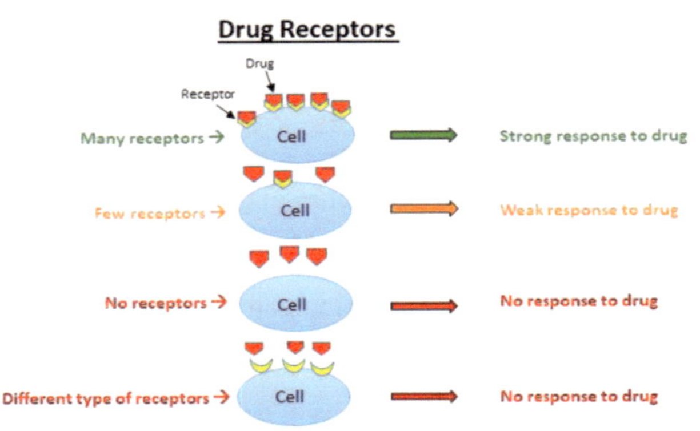

Figure 1.
Patient response relative to drug-receptor interactions and receptor availability.

receptor 2 (HER2) receptor. Some breast cancers make too much HER2 and this extra HER2 helps the cancer develop and spread. T-DM1 has shown potential activity in this subset of patients in small clinical series because it works by attaching to HER2 on cancerous cells and killing them. In terms of receptor availability, this mean if a patient tumor has a high amount of HER2 (HER2 positive), the doctor may prescribe T-DM1; but if the tumor does not have enough HER2 (HER2 negative), T-DM1 will not work for such a patient [8].

1.1.2 Drug uptake

Some drugs have receptor inside the cells or receptor binding sites on the inside part of the target cell. Therefore these drugs need to be actively taken into the tissues and cells in which they act. The ability and the rate of a cell to uptake the drug is determined by that cell's genetic makeup. The genetic makeup can also affect how quickly some drugs are removed from the cells in which they act and if drugs are pumped out from the cell too quickly, they might not have time to elicit observed effect. Decreased uptake can mean that the drug does not work as well and can cause it to build up in other parts of your body, which can cause problems (refer to **Figure 2** below) [2].

For instance, in the treatment of dyslipidaemia (high cholesterol and/or fats levels in blood) drugs called statins are used to reduce cholesterol from the liver and these drugs are known to cause muscle problems. Intake of simvastatin for the disease requires that the drug be taken up into the liver by the protein encoded by SLCO1B1 gene. Some people have a specific change in this gene that causes less of simvastatin to be taken into the liver. Intake of high doses of simvastatin could lead to build up of the drug in the muscles, causing muscle weakness and pain. Therefore prior to prescribing simvastatin, genetic testing of SLCO1B1 gene to check if simvastatin is the best statin for use is key [9].

1.1.3 Drug breakdown

Genetic factors that influence enzyme levels account for differences in drug breakdown, giving rise to "genetic polymorphisms" in drug metabolism. If the patient breaks the drug down more quickly than most people, the body gets rid of the drug faster and the patient might need more of the drug or a different drug; lesser if the body breaks the drug down more slowly as illustrated in **Figure 3** below.

Metabolic reactions mediated by P450 phase I enzymes typically modify functional groups (–OH, –SH, $-NH_2$, $-OCH_3$) of endogenous and exogenous compounds (drugs), resulting in an alteration of the biological activity of the compound. Phase I enzymes are involved in the metabolism of over 75% of prescription drugs; therefore, polymorphisms in these enzymes may significantly affect blood levels, which in turn may alter response to many drugs [10].

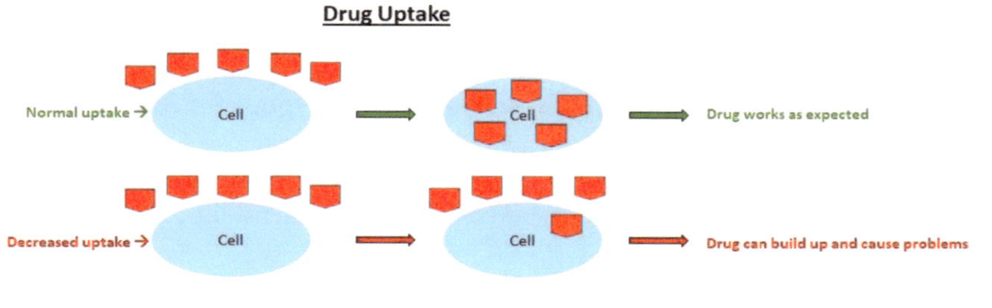

Figure 2.
Differences in drug uptake and potential accumulation leading to toxicity.

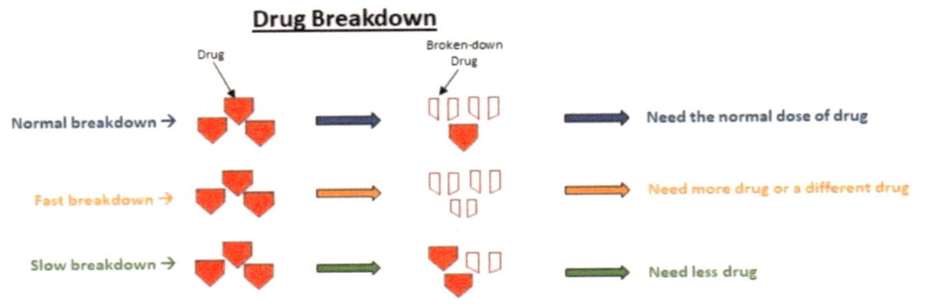

Figure 3.
Rates of drug metabolism.

1.2 The impact of pharmacogenomics on medical treatment

Pharmacogenomics provides a better understanding the reasons behind the differing responses of a drug by individuals. The discovery of genetic variation and its associated response variation to a drug, provide the basis for recommending a drug regimen to an individual patient. Genetic makeup-based prescription, design, and implementation of therapy do not only improve the outcome of treatments, but also reduce the risk of toxicity and other adverse events. Therefore genetic testing promotes a better understanding of individual variations and their effect on drug response, metabolism excretion, toxicity and this will replace the trial-and-error approach of treatment which is a common practice [11]. Pharmacogenomics promote personalized medicine instead.

1.3 Biomarkers and "core" essential drugs

The **Table 1** below is a summary of "core list"essential medicines identified from the 21st WHO EML updated in June 2019 [5] presented against the corresponding biomarkers and therapeutic areas from the USFDA Table of Pharmacogenomic Biomarkers in Drug Labeling updated in June 2020 [6].

2. Clinical pharmacogenomics of the biomarkers and implicated drugs

2.1 Cytochrome p450 isozymes

Polymorphic cytochrome P450 isozymes, CYP2C9, CYP2C19 and CYP2D6 in particular, mediate approximately 40% of P450-oxidative drug metabolism, which makes drug dosing problematic. Generally four genetically different types of individuals have been identified, namely:

1. Poor metabolizers (PMs), who lack the functional enzyme;

2. Intermediary metabolizers (IMs), who are heterozygous for one deficient allele or carry two alleles that cause reduced enxyme activity;

3. Extensive metabolizers (EMs), who have two normal alleles; and

4. Ultrarapid metabolizers (UMs), who have two have multiple gene copies, a trait that is dominantly inherited.

Biomarker	Drug (s)	Therapeutic area
CYB5R	Metoclopramide	Gastroenterology
CYP2B6	Efavirenz	Infectious diseases
CYP2C19	Clopidogrel	Cardiology
	Diazepam	Neurology
	Ethinyloestradiol	Gynaecology
	Omeprazole	Gastroenterology
	Voriconazole	Infectious diseases
CYP2C9	Phenytoin	Neurology
	Warfarin	Hematology
CYP2D6	Amitryptilline	Psychiatry
	Codeine	Anaesthesiology
	Fluoxetine	Psychiatry
	Ondansetron	Gastroenterology
	Risperidone	Psychiatry
	Quinine	Infectious diseases
DYPD	fluorouracil	Oncology
G6PD	Ascorbic acid	Gastroenterology
	Ceftriaxone	Infectious diseases
	Chloroquine	Infectious diseases
	Erythromycin	Infectious diseases
	Nitrofurantoin	Infectious diseases
	Potassium chloride	Gastroenterology
	Primaquine	Infectious diseases
	Sulfasalazine	Gastroenterology
	Sodium chloride	Gastroenterology
	Sulfadiazine	Infectious diseases
	Tetracaine	Anaesthesiology
	Quinine	Infectious diseases
	Sulfamethoxazole	Infectious diseases
	Trimethoprim	Infectious diseases
	Dapsone	Infectious diseases
HLA-B	Abacavir	Infectious diseases
	Carbamazepine	Psychiatry
IFNL3 (IL28B)	Daclatasavir	Infectious diseases
	Dasabuvir	Infectious diseases
	Ledipasvir	Infectious diseases
	Ombitasvir	Infectious diseases
	Paritaprevir	Infectious diseases
	Ritonavir	Infectious diseases
	Sofosbuvir	Infectious diseases

Biomarker	Drug (s)	Therapeutic area
Nonspecific (Congenital Methemoglobinemia)	Dapsone	Infectious diseases
	Lidocaine	Anaesthesiology
Nonspecific (Genetic Susceptibility to Malignant Hyperthermia)	Isoflurane	Anaesthesiology
Nonspecific (NAT)	Sulfamethoxazole	Infectious diseases
	Trimethoprim	Infectious diseases
	Hydralazine	Cardiology
	Sodium Nitrite	Toxicology
POLG	Valproic acid	Neurology
PROC1	Warfarin	Hematology
	Estradiol	Gynaecology
SERPINC1 (Antithrombin III)	Progesterone	Gynaecology
UGT1A1	Dolutegravir	Infectious diseases
	Raltegravir	Infectious diseases
VKORC1	Warfarin	Hematology

Table 1.
Biomarkers, "core" essential drugs and their therapeutic areas.

Polymorphism of cytochrome P450 metabolizing enzymes has the greatest effect on inter individual variability of drug response. These polymorphisms affect the response of individuals to drugs used in the treatment of diseases not limited to cardiology, hematology, neurology, psychiatry, gynaecology, gastroenterology, anaesthesiology and infectious diseases [12].

The effect on CYP2C9 on warfarin dosing has been evident. Individuals who are heterozygous for a *2 allele and *3 allele of CYP2C9 would require, on average, a 21% and 34% lower daily dose of warfarin for maintenance, respectively; than homozygous wild-type patients, and individuals who are homozygous for the *2 allele or the *3 allele require a 60–75% lower dose of warfarin than homozygous wild-type patients [13].

CYP2D6 is responsible for the metabolism of most psychoactive drugs, including the tricyclic antidepressants and the dosage required corresponds closely with the CYP2D6 phenotype. The kinetics of nortriptyline is dependent on the number of active CYP2D6 genes and the dosage required to reach the same plasma levels varies from 30 to 50 mg in PMs to 500 mg in UMs [14].

The majority of phenytoin metabolism is done by CYP2C9 and effective dosing of phenytoin is highly linked to the CYP2C9 genotype. Several examples of adverse effects of phenytoin, including CNS intoxication and other neurological symptoms, have been described in patients with defective CYP2C9 alleles following phenytoin treatment [15].

Dosing with proton pump inhibitors to reach a therapeutic drug plasma concentration highly depends on the CYP2C19 phenotype. A study conducted using a low dose omeprazole (20 mg) to treat ulcers, revealed very low cure rates in EMs (25%), higher in IMs (50%) and complete in PMs (100%), illustrating the necessity of higher plasma levels for effective treatment [16].

CYP2B6 polymorphisms can affect the pharmacokinetics and therapeutic outcome of anti-HIV agents, such as efavirenz, which is a substrate of CYP2B6. The CYP2B6*6 allele harboring the 516G > T (Q172H) and 785A > G (K262R) was significantly associated with a pronounced decrease in CYP2B6 expression and activity. CYP2B6 genetic polymorphisms markedly influence the metabolism of efavirenz in human liver microsomes [17].

2.2 Cytochrome b5 reductases (CYB5R)

Patients with NADH-cytochrome b5 reductase deficiency, encoded by CYB5R1, CYB5R2, CYB5R3 and CYB5R4 genes, are at an increased risk of developing methemoglobinemia and/or sulfhemoglobinemia when metoclopramide is administered. Additionally, neonates have reduced levels of NADH-cytochrome b5 reductase and prolonged drug clearance, and therefore are also more susceptible to methemoglobinemia [18].

2.3 Non-cytochrome p450 enzymes

2.3.1 Vitamin K epoxide reductase complex subunit 1 (VKORC1)

The wide variation in warfarin dose highlights the heterogeneity amongst patients in therapeutic response to warfarin. A study conducted by Harrington *et al.* demonstrated that a heterozygous 196G → A transition that predicted a Valine-66 Methionine substitution in the VKORC1 polypeptide is the cause of warfarin resistance [19]. VKORC1 polymorphisms can significantly changes pharmacodynamics and maintenance dose requirements for warfarin. Patients with the 1639A (rs992323) and 1173 T (rs9934438) allele require a lower warfarin dose compared with patients with 9041A (rs7294) allele rather need a higher warfarin dose. Incorporating VKORC1 and CYP2C9 genotype information into the warfarin dosing equation holds great promise to select the optimal dose for the individual patient at the start of warfarin therapy [20].

2.3.2 Glucose-6-Phosphate Dehydrogenase (G6PD)

G6PD deficiency is an X-linked genetic disorder with 187 known allelic mutations. G6PD is a critical enzyme in the pentose phosphate pathway. G6PD deficiency exhibits diminished activity in these patients, leading to inadequate production of protective intracellular thiols during oxidative stress. The deficiency makes erythrocytes more vulnerable to oxidative stress and has been associated with neonatal hyperbilirubinemia, acute hemolysis, and chronic nonspherocytic hemolytic anemia [21]. Some drugs should be avoided by all G6PD-deficient patients: these include primaquine, nitrofurantoin, and dapsone; while others like IV ascorbic acid, chloroquine and quinine should be used with caution.

2.3.3 Uridine diphosphate-glucuronosyltransferase 1A1 (UGT1A1)

Dolutegravir (DTG) is metabolized mainly by UGT1A1. Individuals carrying UGT1A1*6 and/or UGT1A1*28 polymorphs were demonstrated to be associated with high DTG trough concentrations, and that carrying UGT1A1*6 and/or UGT1A1*28 alleles might be a risk factor for neuropsychiatric adverse events [22]. HIV-1 infected patients demonstrated significant impact of UGT1A1*28 variant on raltegravir exposure with UGT1A1*28 carriers showing higher raltegravir plasma levels and lower metabolic ration when compared to UGT1A1*1/*1 carriers. This effect appeared to be allele-dose dependent. This pharmacokinetic effect did not correlate with any clinical adverse events or biological abnormalities except for the sensation of fatigue. Some virological failures have been associated with low raltegravir exposure; hence UGT1A1*28 genotyping may still be considered as an interesting tool to improve raltegravir therapy particularly when risk factors for virological failure are present, such as high viral load at baseline, once daily regimen or when raltegravir is used to replace high genetic barrier drug in treatment-exposed patients [23].

2.3.4 Human leukocyte antigen B (HLA-B)

Abacavir-induced hypersensitivity reaction has been associated with the presence of the major histocompatibility complex class I allele HLA-B*5701. A screening test for the HLA-B*5701 allele can assist clinicians to identify patients who are at risk of developing a hypersensitivity reaction to abacavir. Abacavir hypersensitivity reaction affects 5 to 8% of patients and can be observed during the first 6 weeks of antiretroviral therapy [24]. Relatively high incidence of HLA-B*1502 in many Asian populations has resulted in the FDA's decision to recommend testing for all Asians prior to initiating carbamazepine. Han Chinese who have the HLA-B*1502 allele are at a much increased risk of developing Stephen-Johnsons Syndrome/ Toxic Epidermal Necrolysis (SJS/TEN) when exposed to carbamazepine [25].

2.3.5 Interferon Lambda 3 (Interleukin-28B)

Sofosbuvir is a potent nucleotide hepatitis C virus (HCV) Nonstructural protein 5B (NS5B) polymerase inhibitor that is also a P-glycoprotein (encoded by the ABCB1 gene) substrate. Sofosbuvir is metabolized mainly into GS-331007 in the liver. ABCB1 gene (3435 CT/TT and 1236 TT genotypes) are the predictors of GS-331007 concentrations [23]. P-glycoprotein (P-gp) removes chemical toxins and metabolites (including GS-331007) from cells into bile, urine and the intestinal lumen. Alterations in P-gp function may affect the bioavailability, distribution and clearance of many drugs [26]. The genetics of IL28B have played an important role in predicting outcome and toxicity of HCV polymerase inhibitors.

2.3.6 DNA polymerase gamma (POLG)

DNA polymerase gamma (POLG) determines the risk of sodium valproate induced liver toxicity. Rare mutations in POLG, which codes for the mitochondrial DNA polymerase gamma, cause the Alpers-Huttenlocher syndrome (AHS); a neuro-metabolic disorder associated with an increased risk of developing fatal sodium valproate hepatotoxicity [27]. Thus, sequencing the POLG gene remains the best diagnostic test to prevent sodium valproate-induced liver failure and patient death.

2.4 Clotting factors

2.4.1 Protein C, inactivator of coagulation factors Va and VIIIa (PROC, PROC1)

PROC encodes for vitamin K-dependent plasma glycoprotein called Protein C. The protein is cleaved to its active form by the thrombomodulin-thrombin complex. The activated form contains a serine protease domain and functions in degradation of the active forms of coagulation factors V and VIII. Mutations of this gene have been associated with thrombophilia due to protein C deficiency and recurrent venous thrombosis [28].

2.4.2 SERPINC1 (Antithrombin III)

The gene SERPINC1 encodes a serine protease inhibitor named antithrombin III (ATIII). Antithrombin III is the most important coagulation factor inhibitor, and even minor changes in ATIII can significantly alter the risk of thromboembolism. The incidence of ATIII-inherited deficiency is relatively rare in the general population but in patients with thromboembolism, the prevalence of ATIII deficiency ranges from 0.5–5%. Acquired deficiency of ATIII can be found in patients on oral contraceptives (progesterone). In overall, patients with the acquired type of ATIII deficiency are exposed to a high risk of thromboembolism, due to depletion of coagulation factor inhibitor critical to anticoagulation in plasma [29, 30].

2.5 Dihydropyrimidine dehydrogenase (DYPD)

The dihydropyrimidine dehydrogenase, encoded by DPYD gene, is an enzyme that catalyzes the rate-limiting step in fluorouracil metabolism. Genetic variations in the DPYD gene can lead to enzymes with reduced or no activity. Individuals who have at least one copy of a non-functional DPYD variant especially the DPYD*2A or DPYD*13, will not be able to metabolize fluorouracil at normally. As a result, these individuals are at risk of potentially life-threatening toxicity to fluorouracil including bone marrow suppression and neurotoxicity. The prevalence of dihydropyrimidine dehydrogenase partial deficiency is approximately 35%; although it varies in different populations. Complete absence of this enzyme function is often fatal with exposure to 5-FU chemotherapy [31].

2.6 Biomarkers inducing genetic susceptibility to diseases

Younker et al. reported a G6PD deficient 22-month-old baby who suffered Malignant Hyperthermia (MH). They concluded that decreased major antioxidant system activity may cause susceptibility to MH [32]. Altikat et al. found that isoflurane has an inhibitory effect on G6PD activity; thus predisposing anaesthesized patient to developing MH [33]. Malignant hyperthermia is a pharmacogenetic disorder in the regulation of calcium in skeletal muscles which is related to an uninhibited muscle hypermetabolic reaction to potent inhalation agents such as isoflurane.

Methemoglobin is an aberrant form of hemoglobin arising from oxidation of iron in the normal heme molecule from the ferrous form (Fe^{2+}) to the ferric (Fe^{3+}) form. The presence of ferric heme molecules causes a structural change in the hemoglobin molecule, resulting in reduced oxygen-carrying capacity and impaired unloading of oxygen at the tissue; resulting in left shift in the oxygen saturation curve causing functional anemia referred to as methemoglobinemia. While methemoglobinemia can be congenital and should be considered in cyanotic infants, it is more often an adverse medication effect, most commonly related to dapsone use. Dapsone most commonly causes methemoglobin, but other offending drugs include the local anesthetics such as lidocaine [34].

3. Conclusion

There is a correlation between individual genetic makeup and the pharmacological response to drugs. Genetic variation plays a pivotal role in the efficacy and safety of different drugs. Thus gene testing prior to initiating concerned treatment is the best clinical practice that will eliminate the "one size fits all" approach and promote personalized approaches that consider individual genetic makeup in attempt to enhance the efficacy and safety of drugs.

4. Future aspects

The future has that the putting in place proper technologies to perform gene testing in clinical settings will be of great help in individualizing treatment to patients. However, genetic polymorphism varies between populations; therefore further research needs to be done on different populations so that gene testing technologies will focus on respective populations.

Author details

Molungoa Sello
National University of Lesotho, Lesotho

*Address all correspondence to: m.sello@nul.ls

References

[1] National Institute of General Medical Sciences. Pharmacogenomics. [Internet]. 2020. https://www.nigms.nih.gov/education/fact-sheets/Pages/pharmacogenomics.aspx [Accessed: 15-01-2021]

[2] Centers for Disease Control (CDC). Pharmacogenomics: What does it mean for your health? [Internet]. 2020. https://www.cdc.gov/genomics/disease/pharma.htm [Accessed: 15-01-2021]

[3] National Human Genome Research Institute. Pharmacogenomics FAQ. [Internet]. 2020. https://www.genome.gov/FAQ/Pharmacogenomics [Accessed: 15-01-2021]

[4] World Health Organization. Essential medicines. [Internet]. 2021. https://www.who.int/topics/essential_medicines/en/ [Accessed: 15-01-2021]

[5] World Health Organization. WHO Model Lists of Essential Medicines. [Internet]. 2021. https://www.who.int/topics/essential_medicines/en/ [Accessed: 15-01-2021]

[6] United States Food and Drug Administration (USFDA). Table of pharmacogenomic biomarkers in drug labeling. [Internet]. 2020. https://www.fda.gov/media/124784/Download [Accessed: 15-01-2021]

[7] Zastrow M. Drug Receptors & Pharmacodynamics. In: Katzung BG. Basic & Clinical Pharmacology, 14th ed. New York; McGraw-Hill Education: 2018 p. 20-40.

[8] Montermurro F, Delaloge S, Barrios CH, Mint: Trastuzumab emtansine (T-DM1) in patients with HER2-positive metastatic breast cancer and brain metastases: exploratory final analysis of cohort 1 from KAMILLA, a single-arm phase IIIb clinical trial. Annals of Oncology. 2020;31(10): 1350-1358.

[9] Voora D, Shah SH, Spasojevic I, Mint: The SLCO1B1*5 genetic variant is associated with statin induced side sffects. Journal of the American college of cardiology. 2009;54(17): 1609-1616.

[10] Hibma JE, Giacomini KM. Pharmacogenomics. In: Katzung BG. Basic & Clinical Pharmacology, 14th ed. New York; McGraw-Hill Education: 2018 p. 74-88.

[11] Singh DB. The Impact of Pharmacogenomics in Personalized Medicine. In: Current Applications of Pharmaceutical Biotechnology, Switzerland; Springer: 2020 p.369-394.

[12] Ingelman-Sundberg M. Pharmacogenetics of cytochrome P450 and its applications in drug therapy: the past, present and future. TRENDS in pharmacological sciences. 2004;25(4): 193-200.

[13] Takahashi H, Echizen H. Pharmacogenetics of CYP2C9 and inter-individual variability in anticoagulant response to warfarin. The Pharmacogenomics Journal. 2003;3(4):202-14.

[14] Dalén P, Dahl ML, Ruiz ML, Mint: 10-Hydroxylation of nortriptyline in white persons with 0, 1, 2, 3, and 13 functional CYP2D6 genes. Clinical pharmacology & therapeutics. 1998;63(4):444-452.

[15] Lee CR, Goldstein JA, Pieper JA. Cytochrome P450 2C9 polymorphisms: a comprehensive review of the in-vitro and human data. Pharmacogenetics and genomics. 2002;12(3):251-263.

[16] Furuta T, Ohashi K, Kamata T, Mint: Effect of genetic differences in omeprazole metabolism on cure

rates for Helicobacter pylori infection and peptic ulcer. Annals of internal medicine. 1998;129(12):1027-1030.

[17] Desta Z, Saussele T, Ward B, Mint: Impact of CYP2B6 polymorphism on hepatic efavirenz metabolism in vitro. Pharmacogenomics. 2007;8(6):547-558.

[18] PharmGKB®. Annotation of FDA Label for metoclopramide and CYB5R1, CYB5R2,CYB5R3,CYB5R4,G6PD. [Internet]. 2021. https://www.pharmgkb.org/labelAnnotation/PA166105195 [Accessed: 22-01-2021]

[19] Harrington DJ, Underwood S, Morse C, Mint: Pharmacodynamic resistance to warfarin associated with a Val66Met substitution in vitamin K epoxide reductase complex subunit 1. Thromb Haemost. 2005;93(1):23-26.

[20] Owen RP, Gong L, Sagreiya H, Mint: VKORC1 pharmacogenomics summary. Pharmacogenetics and genomics. 2010;20(10):642-644.

[21] Luzzatto L. Hemolytic anemias and anemia due to acute blood loss. In: Longo DL, Fauci AS, Kasper DL, Mint: Harrison's Principles of Internal Medicine. 18th ed, New York: McGraw-Hill; 2012.

[22] Yagura H, Watanabe D, Kushida H, Mint: Impact of UGT1A1 gene polymorphisms on plasma dolutegravir trough concentrations and neuropsychiatric adverse events in Japanese individuals infected with HIV-1. BMC infectious diseases. 2017;17(1):1-8.

[23] Belkhir L, Seguin-Devaux C, Elens L, Mint: Impact of UGT 1 A1 polymorphisms on Raltegravir and its glucuronide plasma concentrations in a cohort of HIV-1 infected patients. Scientific reports. 2018;8(1):1-8.

[24] Cutrell A, Hernandez J, Edwards M, Mint: Clinical risk factors for hypersensitivity reactions to abacavir: retrospective analysis of over 8000 subjects receiving abacavir in 34 clinical trials. In43rd Annual Interscience Conference on Antimicrobial Agents and Chemotherapy 2003:pp. 14-17.

[25] Ferrell PB, McLeod HL. Carbamazepine, HLA-B* 1502 and risk of Stevens–Johnson syndrome and toxic epidermal necrolysis: US FDA recommendations. Pharmacogenomics. 2008; 9(10): 1543-1546.

[26] Cusato J, De Nicolò A, Boglione L, Mint: Pharmacogenetics of the anti-HCV drug sofosbuvir: a preliminary study. Journal of Antimicrobial Chemotherapy. 2018;73(6): 1659-1664.

[27] Matheny CJ, Lamb MW, Brouwer KL, Mint: Pharmacokinetic and pharmacodynamic implications of P-glycoprotein modulation. Pharmacotherapy: The Journal of Human Pharmacology and Drug Therapy. 2001;21(7):778-796.

[28] Stewart JD, Horvath R, Baruffini E, Mint: Polymerase γ gene POLG determines the risk of sodium valproate-induced liver toxicity. Hepatology. 2010;52(5):1791-1796.

[29] NCBI Reference Sequence Database. PROC protein C, inactivator of coagulation factors Va and VIIIa [*Homo sapiens* (human)]. [Internet]. 2021. https://www.ncbi.nlm.nih.gov/gene?Db=gene&Cmd=DetailsSearch&Term=5624 [Accessed: 25-01-2021]

[30] Găman AM, Găman GD. Deficiency of Antithrombin III (AT III)-case report and review of the literature. Current health sciences journal. 2014;40(2):141-143.

[31] Dean L, Kane M. Fluorouracil therapy and DPYD genotype. Medical Genetics Summaries. 2021:1-18

[32] Younker D, De Vore MA, Hartlage P. Malignant hyperthermia and glucose-6-phosphate dehydrogenase deficiency. Anesthesiology. 1984;60(6):601-603.

[33] Altikat S, Çiftçi M, Buyukokuroglu ME. In vitro effects of some anesthetic drugs on enzymatic activity of human red blood cell glucose 6-phosphate dehydrogenase. Polish journal of pharmacology. 2002;54(1):67-72.

[34] Mansouri A, Lurie AA. Methemoglobinemia. American journal of hematology. 1993;42(1):7-12.

Section 4

In Silico Studies on Pharmacogenetics

Chapter 9

In Silico Studies on Pharmacokinetics and Neuroprotective Potential of $^{25}Mg^{2+}$: Releasing Nanocationites - Background and Perspectives

Valentin V. Fursov, Ilia V. Fursov, Alexander A. Bukhvostov, Aleksander G. Majouga and Dmitry A. Kuznetsov

Abstract

Sharp blood circulation disorders are known for their capability to promote such abundant and hardly treatable pathologies as myocardium infarction and the ischemic brain stroke ("insult"). Noteworthy, the stroke — related brain tissue metabolic damages involve an essential ATP deplete clash along with a suppression of brain specific nucleotide — associated kinases and ATP synthase, both Mg^{2+} — dependent complex enzyme "machineries". This itself makes the latter's a legitimate target for some advanced pharmaceuticals as long as the drug — induced overstimulation of corresponding enzymatic activity is the case. Thus, magnetic isotope effects (MIE) of the nuclear spin possessing paramagnetic $^{25}Mg^{2+}$ ions might modulate the brain creatine kinase, alfa-glycerophosphate kinase and pyruvate kinase catalytic activities in a way of a remarkable ATP hyperproduction required to compensate the hypoxia caused acute metabolic breakdown. To realize the Magnesium-25 pharmacological potential, a low-toxic amphiphilic cationite nanoparticles were introduced lately. Particularly, the Magnesium — releasing porphyrin-fullerene nanoadduct (cyclohexyl-C60-porphyrin, PMC16) has been proposed to meet expectations dealing with a targeted delivery of $^{25}Mg^{2+}$ towards the brain ischemia surrounding areas. In order to optimize a multi-step $[^{25}Mg^{2+}]_4$PMC16 preclinical trial scenario, the In Silico algorithms are to be developed and analyzed. In this study, these algorithms are in a focus with a special emphasize on a novel combination of slightly modified Gompertzian equation systems and a non-Markov population dynamics concept. This In Silico approach takes into account some literature-available patterns of brain hypoxia pathogenesis, the resulted simulation model could be considered as a promising tool for further research on experimental nanopharmacology of the ischemic stroke.

Keywords: Magnetic isotope effects, brain ischemia disorders, hypoxia, fullerene— porphyrin nanoparticles, In Silico pharmacokinetic algorithms

1. Introduction. Formulation of the problem

Research in the field of development of promising drugs for the treatment of ischemic stroke based on nanoparticle carriers of cations of paramagnetic isotopes of divalent metals is at an early stage. Such studies are compounded by the lack of descriptions of relevant mathematical models of ischemic stroke in scientific literature, as well as drug-specific models of the pharmacokinetics of targeted delivery of PMC16 nanoparticles. All this is required for the development of In Silico instruments for preclinical and clinical studies of the neuroprotective potential of $[^{25}Mg^{2+}]_4$PMC16 in the treatment of ischemic stroke [1–4] (**Figure 1**).

Creation of In Silico - algorithms for optimization of multistage scenarios of preclinical trials of $[^{25}Mg^{2+}]_4$PMC16 in experimental nanopharmacology of ischemic stroke represents a completely new, complex, innovative and challenging interdisciplinary problem.

Speaking of the direct and clear practical benefits which are supposed to be gained from the appropriate use of mathematical modeling in specifying the plan of preclinical anti-hypoxia medicines research, this requirement is undoubtedly essential for optimizing this plan. Notably, an applied pharmacological potential of such a peculiar *In Silico* simulation approach might be taken as a "hopeful pullout" for coming up with a novel element in a preclinical trial strategy for prevention of metabolic breakdown in brain ischemia and/or correction based on the administration of paramagnetic bivalent metal isotopes released and delivered by amphiphilic nano-cationites belonging to the superfamily of PMC16 (C60-porphyrin) nanoparticles [5].

Noteworthy, a so-called "sovereign trend" in computational modeling of pharmacological processes within the current preclinical trial paradigm has already made a significant impact on preclinical trial design in experimental neurology and neuropharmacology [6–8]. This correlates with the PubMed statistics showing a remarkable increase in the number of publications on the above-specified issue [6].

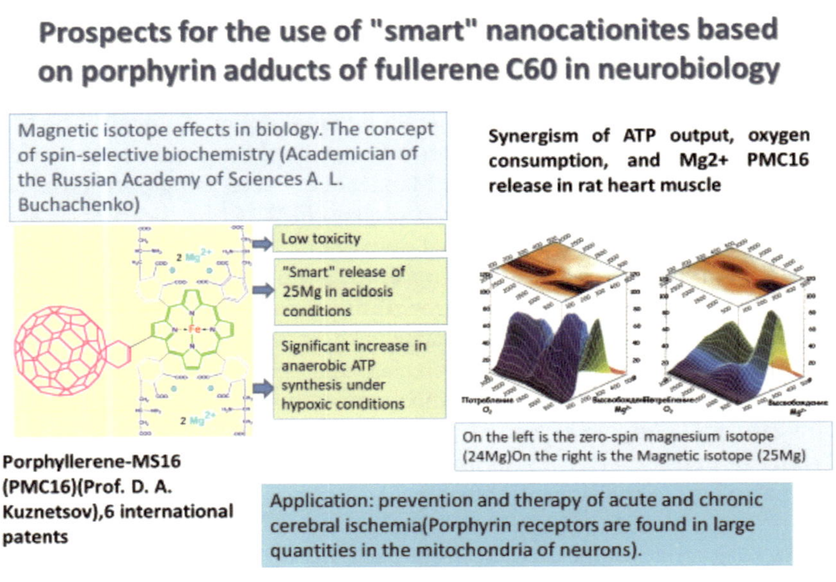

Figure 1.
Prospects for the use in neurobiology of "smart" nano-cationites based on porphyrin adducts of fullerene C60.

2. Methods

Simulation of processes occurring in biological objects and systems is necessary to optimize algorithms for preclinical and clinical studies in pharmacology. These tasks are solved using *in vitro, in vivo, In Silico* models. Modeling is one of the leading research methods of this kind. The variety of processes in a living organism is so great that it is almost impossible to get a detailed and complete understanding of the behavior of a living system. In view of this, the development of new treatment methods, diagnosis, pharmacy, etc., requires the modeling of objects of appropriate research. Any type of modeling consists of replacing the investigated object (process, phenomenon) with a model, which is a semblance of a real object (process, phenomenon). At the same time, such an object representing the model is consciously perceived as simplified. However, it is vital that it retains the main, most essential properties for research, which are available for a real object (system, process, phenomenon).

Modeling is a method in which the study of its model replaces the study of a complex object (process, phenomenon). Accordingly, such an object (process, phenomenon) itself, which resembles the real object, but has been deliberately simplified, is called a *model*.

Any scientific research method, including both theoretical and empirical, is based on the idea of modeling.

In this work, we will adhere to the classical algorithm for constructing mathematical models adopted in biophysics.

The main stages of modeling can be summarized as follows:

1. Primary collection of information about the object of modeling: about its properties, processes occurring in it, patterns of behavior under various external conditions.

2. Formulation of the problem. The goal of the study and its main tasks are formulated. It is determined what new knowledge should be obtained after the research has been conducted.

3. Substantiation of basic assumptions. It is necessary to determine the characteristics of the object that are insignificant for solving the research problem, which can be neglected.

4. Creating a model, researching it.

5. Checking the relevance of the model to the object under study.

3. General task structure

The difficulty lies not only in the fact that in the domestic and foreign literature, there are no relevant mathematical models of ischemic stroke, and they need to be created almost from scratch, but also within the problem itself, which arises from the necessity not only to develop but also to align mathematical models of several processes mutually:

1. The process of necrosis of brain tissue as a result of ischemia and related phenomena (apoptosis, toxicosis, edema, etc.) in the absence of pharmacotherapy;

2. Pharmacokinetics (i.e., delivery) of the $[^{25}Mg^{2+}]_4PMC16$ drug to the desired area of the brain and distribution throughout the tissue;

3. Model of the process of the effect of the drug $[^{25}Mg^{2+}]_4PMC16$ on the synthesis of ATP and the prolongation of the life cycle of cells, which are subjected to hypoxic conditions, but have not lost their viability;

4. The recovery process (reperfusion, [neuro]glialisation, regeneration) of the functions of living ischemic cells as a consequence of the pharmacotherapy of ischemic stroke with the drug $[^{25}Mg^{2+}]_4PMC16$.

5. Phagocytosis.

6. Other processes.

The general structure of the problem is shown in (**Figure 2**).

At the same time, the *In Silico* development process is implemented in several stages:

1. Formation of a hypothesis and a general structural model *In Silico*.

2. Acceptance of initial constraints and simplifications.

3. Formation of hypotheses and primary models of processes.

4. Mathematical modeling of individual processes.

5. Combining mathematical models of individual processes into a system of differential equations.

6. Search for optimal solutions to the system of differential equations (*In Silico* level I).

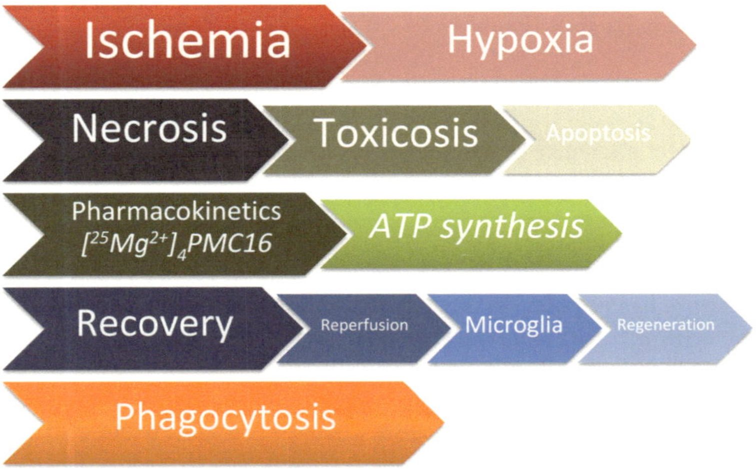

Figure 2.
General structure of the task of developing In Silico *pharmacokinetics and neuroprotective potential of fullerene-porphyrin nano-cationites carrying* $^{25}Mg^{2+}$ *in relation to the pathogenesis of ischemic stroke.*

7. *In Silico* level II development: algorithmization, IT programming, debugging, testing.

8. Use of level II *In Silico* for prediction and simulation of *in vivo*.

9. Raising accuracy, development, improvement.

10. Development of "smart" *In Silico* level III based on *artificial intelligence neural networks*: Design of neural network architecture, debugging, training, testing.

11. Use of "smart" *In Silico* level III as a predictive tool for preclinical trials.

12. Laying the foundations of smart *In Silico* level IV architecture as a predictive tool for clinical trials.

4. Mathematical modeling of ischemic stroke. Hypothesis formation

Mathematical modeling of ischemic stroke is a complex task in itself. Several pathogenetic subtypes (atherothrombotic, cardioembolic, lacunar, hemodynamic and microcirculatory) have been highlighted. Accordingly, the mechanisms of occurrence and development of the disease also differ. All this significantly complicates the modeling of the development of this disease at the level of hypotheses and primary algorithms laid down in the *In Silico* process. This nosology of ischemic stroke complicates approaches to the formation of primary algorithms for the process of occurrence and course of ischemic stroke, as well as solving problems of mathematical formalization.

It is customary to distinguish 4 stages [9] of ischemic stroke (**Figure 3**):

1. Terminated (3–5 days)

2. Most acute (7–10 days)

3. Acute (up to 1 month)

4. Early recovery (up to 6 months)

5. Late recovery (from 6 months to 1 year)

6. Long-term (over 1 year)

Of these, the acute phase is characterized by the most severe course and high mortality, which is why the study of patterns of the disease in the acute phase (first five days of the disease) is the most significant. During this period, the right therapeutic tactics can bring the maximum result. During this period, the drug $[^{25}Mg^{2+}]_4$PMC16 should have the maximum positive effect on the dynamics of the course of the disease.

In the development process *in silico*, we will build on the simplest concepts of the course of the disease, introducing some assumptions and simplifications. According to the need to improve the model, these simplifications will subsequently be removed or replaced by more complex designs. Then the problem of merging the models of the various processes as mentioned earlier into a single structure needs to be solved.

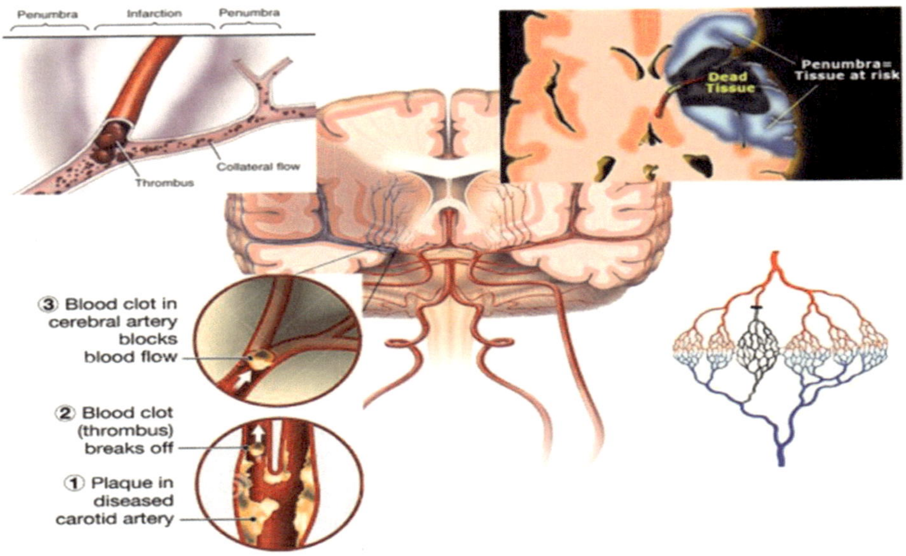

Figure 3.
Graphic model of ischemic stroke, the development of ischemic penumbra and the spread of the damaged brain tissue due to ischemia and blockage of the vascular bed branch.

Based on this, we will simplify the growth of an ischemic stroke as a process of necrotic death of cells of normal brain tissue caused by a stop in the blood supply to its part due to blockage of a part of the vascular bed that feeds the brain. Consequently, hypoxia begins to develop in the area of the brain, the blood supply of which was carried out from the clogged vascular network. As a result of hypoxia, cells that lack oxygen begin to die off gradually. A process of necrosis of this part of the brain's tissues takes place (**Figure 3**).

The process of necrotic cell death is stretched out in time. For this reason, there is a transition region between the infarct nucleus and healthy tissue (ischemic penumbra), in which the functions of the cells are disrupted, but they remain viable. It is vital to note that penumbra cells' death is reversible and progresses more slowly than in the infarct nucleus, within a few hours [10]. This "therapeutic window" (at least 3–6 hours) provides time for diagnosis and treatment measures aimed at restoring nerve cells, limiting the area of damage and reducing neurological consequences.

Thus, in order to solve the general problem: the *in silico* development of the neuroprotective potential of $[^{25}Mg^{2+}]_4$PMC16 nanoparticles, it is necessary to develop *in silico* of ischemic stroke and combine this model with the pharmacokinetics of $[^{25}Mg^{2+}]_4$PMC16 as a drug. At the same time, it is necessary to consider the particularities of targeting (targeted delivery) of $[^{25}Mg^{2+}]_4$PMC16 nanoparticles in the infarction zone, more precisely in the area of ischemic penumbra.

5. Acceptance of initial restrictions and simplifications

Starting the mathematical modeling of ischemic stroke at the cellular level, we will accept a number of assumptions and simplifications, namely:

1. We consider the brain to be homogeneous in composition, structure and cell type. Cell differentiation is neglected;

2. We do not consider any other causes of cell death other than necrosis as a result of hypoxia;

3. We do not consider the processes of removing the decay products of dead cells and toxins that occur in the process of brain activity;

4. We do not take into account the consequences of brain tissue necrosis, such as edema, an increase in the volume of necrotizing tissue, leading, in particular, to a spike in intracranial pressure, deformation of brain structure, etc.

5. We will assume that brain volume and the number of its cells before, after and during the development of a stroke remain unchanged;

6. We will assume that there is a certain "point of no return" for brain cells in the process of hypoxia, after which the process of cell restoration (regeneration) is not possible. This factor affects the size of the ischemic penumbra zone;

7. We will assume that during the period considered in silico, the general blood supply to the brain and the body as a whole does not stop (the patient does not die);

8. We will assume that no outside interference (both therapeutic and surgical) is carried out in the body during the period under consideration.

9. In this way, the general model of the dynamics of the development of ischemic stroke in time will look as follows, presented below (**Figure 4**):

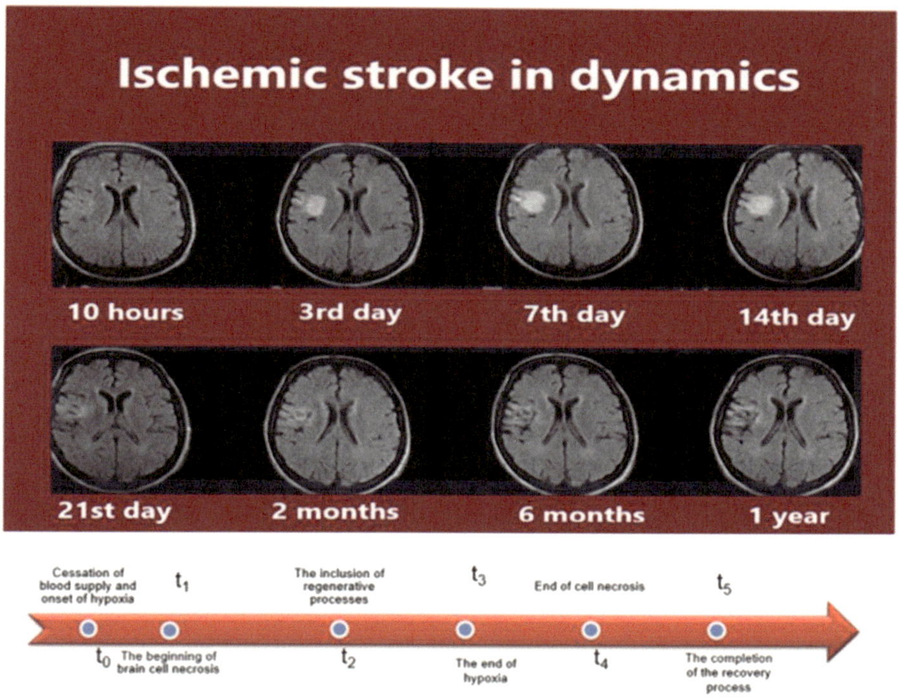

Figure 4.
Time model of progression of ischemic stroke. In the figure: t_0 is the moment when blood supply stops and hypoxia begins, t_1 is the onset of cell necrosis, t_2 is the start of recovery processes, t_2 is the moment of cessation of brain cell death, t_3 is the moment when hypoxia ends (blood supply is restored), t_4 is the end of cell necrosis, t_5 is the moment of completion of the post-stroke recovery process.

6. Formation of hypotheses and primary models of processes

Then, in light of the assumptions made, for the purposes of mathematical modeling, the hypothesis of the scenario of ischemic stroke progression will look in the following manner.

Until time t_0 (pre-stroke phase), the brain functions normally, the blood supply is not disrupted. At time t_0 instantaneous (additional) cessation of blood supply occurs, and the process of necrotization of the brain tissue begins. We believe cell death in hypoxia is also stretched over time and occurs in stages. That is, up to a specific time period t_1, the cell is still capable of recovery, and we can talk about the existence of a "point of no return", after which cell recovery is impossible. We will take this into account later. At time t_2 recovery processes in the body are activated, due to the entry of blood supply from the brain area that has not undergone necrosis. Thus, we can talk about the presence of two "counter" processes in the model of ischemic stroke: the process of dying (necrotization) of cells and the process of restoring the functions of brain cells (**Figure 5**).

Based on this, we can distinguish the following phases of ischemic stroke:

1. Pre-stroke phase, $t \leq t_0$,

2. The phase of brain cell death (necrotic phase), $t_0 \leq t \leq t_4$;

3. Brain cell recovery phase, $t_2 \leq t \leq t_3$;

4. Post-stroke phase, $t \geq t_5$.

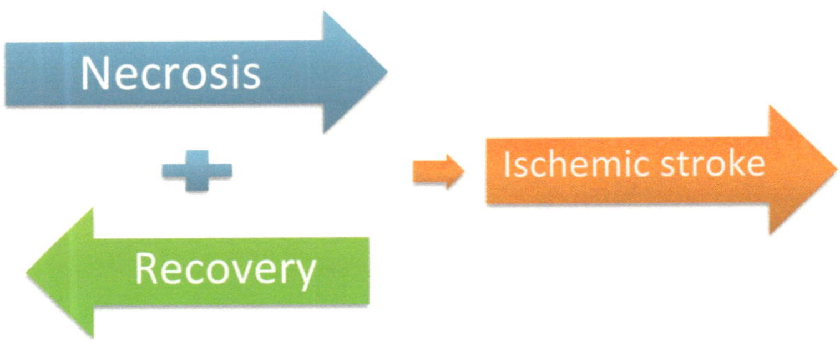

Figure 5.
Counter processes and the resulting process of ischemic stroke growth.

7. Mathematical modeling of individual processes

Now, we can write in general algebraic form the first simple equation, which we will call the "hypoxia equation", describing the amount of GM tissue that has undergone hypoxia at time $\Delta t = t - t_0$, taking $t_0 = 0$ as the starting point of the hypoxia period. ($\Delta t = t$):

$$Q_g = v_g * t \tag{1}$$

Where Q_g – the amount of GM tissue that has undergone hypoxia,
v_g – specific rate of hypoxia (death) of the brain tissue,
t – time elapsed since the end of the blood supply to the brain area.

In this case, the amount of necrotizing tissue can be represented as its volume V, mass m, or the number of dead N_d cells. At the same time, the structure of the formula will not change. Analogously to formula Eq. (1), we write down the necrosis formula for the number of dead N_d cells:

$$N_d(t) = \delta * t \quad (2)$$

Where $N_d(t)$ – the number of dead cells since the end of the blood supply,
δ – specific rate of cell necrosis (death),
t – the time elapsed since the end of the blood supply.
Or, in differential notation:

$$\frac{dN_d(t)}{dt} = \delta N_d \quad (3)$$

Similarly, let us write in differential form the formula for the regeneration of brain cells in the ischemic zone.

$$\frac{dN_R(t)}{dt} = \alpha N_R \quad (4)$$

Where $N_R(t)$ – number of recovered cells,
α – the specific rate of cell repair.
Under our assumptions, the conservation law (balance formula) will look like this:

$$N_{tot} = N_n(t) + N_g(t) \quad (5)$$

Where N_{tot} – the total number of brain cells,
$N_n(t)$ – the number of living normal cells not exposed to hypoxia,
$N_g(t)$ – the number of hypoxidated cells and those at different stages of necrosis (dying).

Assuming that the volume of the brain does not change, and due to the assumption of its homogeneity and the absence of processes for removing dead and damaged cells, the number of brain cells also does not change, we can write:

$$N_{tot} = const \quad (6)$$

It is obvious that the number of hypoxidated cells consists of dead cells that are no longer subject to restoration and regenerated cells, since the processes of dying and restoration in the population of hypoxidated cells proceed simultaneously.

$$N_g(t) = N_d(t) + N_R(t) \quad (7)$$

Then equation Eq. (7) can be rewritten as follows:

$$N_n(t) + N_d(t) + N_R(t) = const \quad (8)$$

Based on our assumptions, and considering that:

$$N_{tot} = \rho * m \quad (9)$$

Where ρ – cell density per unit of brain mass, m is brain mass.
The balance formula Eq. (8) can be rewritten as follows:

$$N_n(t) + N_d(t) + N_R(t) = \rho m \quad (10)$$

where in our assumptions $\rho, m = const$.

The derived formula will be useful in the future for clarifying *In Silico* by *in vitro* because in biological models and in humans, the volume and mass of the brain, and therefore the number of brain cells, are different. If no distinction is made between healthy normal cells, which have not been exposed to hypoxia, and restored cells, their sum, i.e. the number of functioning cells, can be designated as $N(t)$. Then the balanced equation will take the following form:

$$N(t) = \rho m - N_d(t) \tag{11}$$

Let us consider a spatial model of progression of necrosis and restoration of brain tissue in the process of hypoxia (**Figure 6**), where we distinguish 3 fundamentally different areas:

Typically, the blood supply to a particular area of the brain is carried out from all sides via the branched vascular network that runs through the brain from the arteries. In case of a local stop of blood supply, the brain will be fed through the active vascular branches located on the periphery of the hypoxic zone. Thus, the cells closest to the focus of the stroke will experience the greatest shortage of blood supply (the focus of the stroke), and the cells located on the periphery will be exposed to the opposite effect (ischemic penumbra).

So, we can imagine that the wave of necrotization, i.e. area 3 (**Figure 6**), from the moment of local blood supply failure (the beginning of hypoxia), spreads from the focus of the stroke (the place of blockage of the vascular bed) to the periphery. The recovery process goes in the opposite direction: from the periphery to the center of ischemia. After a short period of time after a local stop of blood circulation and the occurrence of hypoxia, necrotization of brain tissue begins. This area of necrotization, expanding, capturing more and more arrays of healthy cells, quickly spreads to the periphery until it meets the area that receives sufficient nutrition from the vascular branches that are not affected by the stroke. Meanwhile, during the development of a stroke, the body starts the recovery processes, increasing the blood supply to the healthy branch. At some point, the "necrotizing wave", which can be called the "stroke front", reaches the brain's area that receives sufficient blood supply from the neighboring unclogged vascular branches. By this time, adaptive processes have already been activated in the body, and through the neighboring non-clogged vascular branches, an increased blood supply is carried out, compared with the norm, sufficient to restore the functions of the brain tissue in the nearby ischemic penumbra. Here, the functions of the cells that are still capable of this restoration are restored. These cells are put back into operation. In this zone, the recovery process

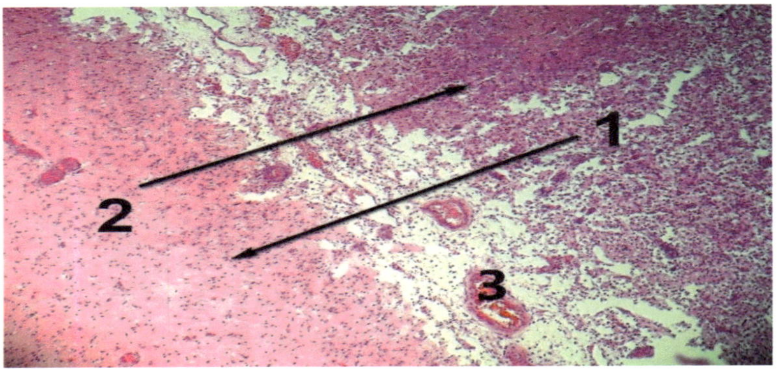

Figure 6.
Brain tissue at the border of the hypoxic zone and the normal zone. Area of normal tissue that has not undergone hypoxia (normal area); 2. Area of dead tissue (area of necrosis); 3. Area of "semi-dead" tissue (ischemic penumbra).

begins to dominate over the necrotic one, and the "stroke front" begins to move in the opposite direction (to the focus of the stroke) under the influence of the recovery process. This recovery process is carried out in the ischemic penumbra until the cells capable of recovery are completely exhausted. This process affects all cells for which recovery is still possible. The cells that have finally died are phagocytized, and their remains are removed from the body through the active vascular networks. The released space is filled with connective or adipose tissue.

This complex process can be considered as two opposite "counter" processes: the process of necrosis and the process of recovery. As mentioned earlier, the recovery process is oppositely directed to the process of necrosis and passes with some delay in time.

They can be represented on average as one, a process that is carried out with a certain specific variable total speed, which consists of the specific speeds of necrotization and recovery.

We can write this circumstance as the sum of the corresponding functions as:

$$\varepsilon(t) = \alpha(t) + \delta(t) \tag{12}$$

Then, the differential equation Eq. (3) is transformed into the following form:

$$\frac{dN_d(t)}{dt} = \varepsilon N_d \tag{13}$$

Where $\varepsilon(t)$ – the specific total speed of the ischemic stroke process, is a rather complex function of many variables.

By rewriting equation Eq. (13) in the form:

$$dN_d(t) = \varepsilon N_d dt \tag{14}$$

The solution of this equation in general form can be obtained by integrating over t in the range $[t_0, t]$:

$$N_d\ (t) = \int_{t_0}^{t} \varepsilon N_d dt \tag{15}$$

At $\varepsilon = const$, which can be understood as the average specific rate of development of necrosis in stroke. The trivial solution to this equation for $N = N_{0,}$ is the exponent:

$$N_d(t) = N_0 e^{\varepsilon t}\ (t \geq 0) \tag{16}$$

Where $N_{0,}$ – the number of brain cells that have undergone hypoxia.

In the case of $\varepsilon < 0$ formula Eq. (17) represents a specific case of a process where necrosis dominates, and eventually, all brain cells that have undergone hypoxia die. In this case, the formula, which we obtained generally reflects the dynamics of necrosis, which leads to the complete death of the population of brain cells, coinciding with the population dynamics according to Malthus (**Figure** 7).

Furthermore, substituting the obtained formula Eq. (16) into the balance equation Eq. (11), we have:

$$N(t) = \rho m - N_0 e^{\varepsilon t} (t \geq 0) \tag{17}$$

Where $N(t)$ – the number of living, functioning (including cells that have undergone hypoxia, but have regained their functions) brain cells during the course of an ischemic stroke,

ρ – brain cells density,

m – brain mass,

N_0 – the number of brain cells that underwent hypoxia during the $[t_0, t]$ course of ischemic stroke,

ε – the specific average rate of ischemic stroke during the period from the beginning of hypoxia to recovery.

The resultant formula is a level I mathematical model obtained with the maximum simplification of the process of ischemic stroke. For large $\varepsilon > 0$ it has no biological meaning. For small positive $\varepsilon \geq 0$, $\varepsilon \to 0$, it exponentially approaches from the value of N_0 to the value of ρm, i.e. it mainly describes the recovery process after the acute phase of an ischemic stroke. The model does not describe the initial phase of an ischemic stroke in sufficient detail, resulting from the simplification made when obtaining the formula (17). Additionally, the model does not clearly express the phases of ischemic stroke development.

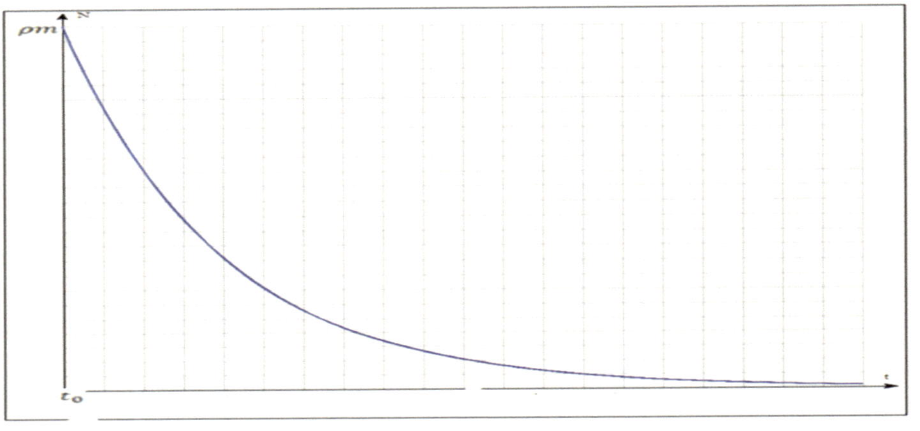

Figure 7.
Model graph of brain cell necrosis.

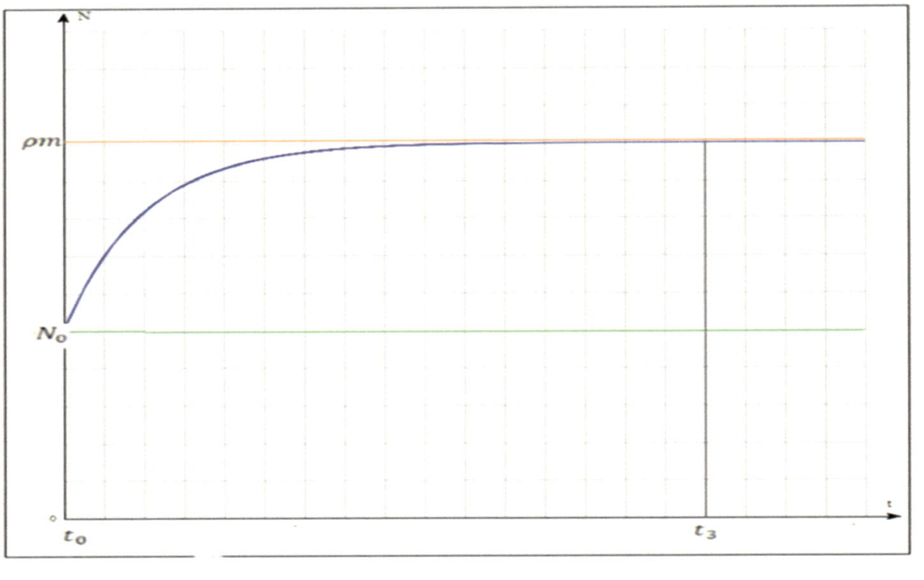

Figure 8.
Graph of the growth of ischemic stroke according to the mathematical model of the first level.

Accordingly, in the most simplified form, we have obtained a mathematical model of level I, which reflects the essence and the general dynamics of ischemic stroke in borderline conditions, but does not take into account many parameters and, accordingly, does not have the required predictive accuracy. According to the level I model, the graph of the development of ischemic stroke is demonstrated in (**Figure 8**).

Further improvement of the mathematical model of ischemic stroke will require the addition and solution of a system of differential equations, the number of which will correspond to the number of input variables. In such cases, you usually have to rely on approximate solutions.

To optimize the multistage scenario of preclinical trials of $[^{25}Mg^{2+}]_4$PMC16, it is necessary to further develop the obtained model and combine it with the pharmacokinetic model of targeted delivery of $[^{25}Mg^{2+}]_4$PMC16 NPs to the hypoxidated area of the brain at the border of healthy and necrotized tissues, for which it is necessary to refine and analyze the *In Silico* algorithms.

8. Combining mathematical models of individual processes into a system of differential equations

Let us detail the pathogenesis model of ischemic stroke and describe the hypothesis of the process at the cellular level in more detail. The previously used simplified model of ischemic stroke pathogenesis reduced death of brain cells from ischemia only to necrosis from hypoxia and did not take into account other factors of the process.

Let us modify the biological model as it was done in [11, 12] the model of brain cell (neurons, astrocytes and other glial cells) death, which takes into account both of the main mechanisms of cell death - apoptosis and necrosis. Nutrient deficiency promotes cell death programs initiation if the level of damage reaches a certain threshold value called D_0. At the present stage of research, we assume that with severe damage, apoptotic or necrotic variants of cell death can be realized with equal probability. The cells that die due to ischemia and subsequent intoxication initiate the immune system's response. First of all, the body's own defenders of nerve cells located in the brain, microglia, are activated, which can ingest (phagocytosis) the decay products, thereby participating in the removal of the destruction products and preventing the escalation of the inflammatory reaction. Activation of microglia prepares them for a state of readiness for phagocytosis and the synthesis of cytokines- specific proteins that coordinate the actions of cells of the immune system. Cytokines cause the accumulation of adhesion molecules in the vicinity of the damage, which promote the attachment (adhesion) of white blood cells traveling in the bloodstream to the endothelium of the blood vessel and their migration through the endothelium to brain cells. As a result, white blood cells overcome the hemato-encephalic barrier characteristic of a healthy body - a physiological mechanism that is designed to regulate the penetration into the brain of various substances introduced from the outside or circulating in the blood, in order to maintain the constancy of the physiological and physicochemical state of the brain. Thus, the cell adhesion molecules initiate the movement of white blood cells into the damaged area. It is known that neutrophils, the most numerous group of small white blood cells, as well as monocytes-macrophages, which are the largest white blood cells, play the main role in phagocytosis. Microglial cells, monocytes-macrophages and neutrophils contribute to the removal of dead apoptotic and necrotic brain cells from the body by phagocytosis. At the same time, activated microglial cells, pro-inflammatory cytokines and neutrophils themselves release toxic substances, which harm intact cells and contribute to the expansion of the brain lesion area [9].

Hence, the mathematical model of the dynamics of brain cell death can be supplemented with the corresponding equations and rewritten in the following form [11, 12]:

$$dH/dt = -\mathrm{DH} \tag{18}$$

$$\mathrm{dN/dt} = \left(1 - p_A\right) \mathrm{DH} - \varepsilon \mathrm{N} \tag{19}$$

$$\mathrm{d}A_s/\mathrm{dt} = p_A \mathrm{DH} - p_A \mathrm{D}\,(\cdot - T_A)\,\mathrm{H}\,(\cdot - T_A) \tag{20}$$

$$\mathrm{d}A_e/\mathrm{dt} = p_A \mathrm{D}\,(\cdot - T_A)\,\mathrm{H}\,(\cdot - T_A) - \varepsilon A_e \tag{21}$$

$$\mathrm{d}M_a/\mathrm{dt} = pM_a(c_A A_e + c_N \mathrm{N})M_i - c_{pro}(M_a/T_{M,1}) \tag{22}$$

$$\begin{aligned} dM_i/dt = -pM_a(c_A A_e + c_N N)M_i + c_{pro} M_a T_{M,1} + \\ (c_{Mi,1}M_i - c_{Mi,2}M_{2i})1_{t>TM,2} - \varepsilon M_i \end{aligned} \tag{23}$$

Where H — relative density of healthy brain cells, N — relative density of necrotic cells, A_s и A_e — relative density of brain cells that started and ended apoptosis, respectively, M_i и M_a — relative density of inactive and active microglial cells; the argument $(\cdot - T_A)$ represents a time delay T_A, corresponding to the characteristic duration of the cell apoptosis process; the sign $1_{t>TM,2}$ also indicates the start of a number of important processes with a delay equal to $T_{M,2}$. In the equations of the mathematical model Eqs. (18)–(23), one of the key roles is played by the values of the specific rate of phagocytosis ε and the specific rate of cell death due to intoxication by decomposition products (inflammation)D, and the latter is different from zero only if the intoxication has reached the established limit level D_0:

$$D = \left[(p_{n,[cy]}C + p_{N,Ln}((L_n/(C_{L_n} + L_n))(N + A_e) + p_{N,N}N) - p_o D_0\right]^+ \tag{24}$$

$$\varepsilon = e_{N,M_a}M_a + e_{N,L_m}L_m + e_{N,L_n}L_n + e_{N,M_i}M_i \tag{25}$$

System (18–23) is supplemented by equations describing the dynamics of inflammation factors:

$$dL_m/dt = c_{Lm}M_{adh}(\cdot - T_{Lm,in}) - p_{dLm}(L_m/T_{Lm}) \tag{26}$$

$$dL_n/dt = c_{Ln}M_{adh}(\cdot - T_{Ln,in}) - p_{dLn}(L_n/T_{Ln}) \tag{27}$$

$$dC/dt = \left(p_{Ma,c}(M_a/M_a + cM_a) + pL_{m.c}(L_m/L_m + cL_m)\right)(N + A_e) - e_{cy}C \tag{28}$$

$$dM_{adh}/dt = \left[p_{Madh,1}C - p_{Madh,2}CM_{adh} - e_{Madh}M_{adh}\right]1_{vessel} \tag{29}$$

Where L_m и L_n — the relative concentration of leukocytes of two types - monocytes-macrophages and neutrophils, respectively, C — relative concentration of cytokines, M_{adh} — the relative density of adhesion molecules. Eq. (29) describes the dynamics of cell adhesion molecules depending on the factors listed in its right-hand side only if the stroke nucleus is located in the vicinity of a blood vessel, and otherwise the density of adhesion molecules remains constant, corresponding to the initial condition. A feature of system (18–29) is the presence of functions with lagging arguments in the right-hand sides of the equations, where the lag $T_{Lm,n}$ and $T_{Ln,in}$, as well as T_A, is due to biomedical considerations. The initial data for the components of the solution to the problem on the time interval $t \in [-\tau, 0]$

(where $\tau = \max(T_A, T_{Lm,in}, T_{Ln,in})$), preceding the onset of the disease are set corresponding to the healthy state: the relative density of healthy cells $H(t) = 1$ and inactive microglia $M_i(t) = 1$, the values of the remaining variables of the problem are assumed to be zero; to simulate a stroke at $t = 0$ a given part of healthy cells (up to 40%) passes into necrotic and / or cells that have entered apoptosis.

Obviously, the mathematical description's complexity will increase in proportion to the number of input variables and the increase in the number of differential equations. Simultaneously, the contribution of each of the new variables or a new differential equation describing the process under consideration at this stage is difficult to predict. In contrast, the entire set of processes accompanying ischemic stroke has not yet been sufficiently studied and described in the literature to be modeled in such detail.

9. Alternative ways of modeling ischemic stroke

At the same time, there are various models of population dynamics, which are used both in biology and in ecology and medicine while having sufficiently high reliability of the mathematical description of processes. Considering that any model is only a semblance of the original and the task of a complete repetition of a real object by a model is never set. Based on the existing models describing population dynamics, it seems possible to select the appropriate one and modify it for the tasks at hand. One of the variants of this approach is to use the modified Gompertz Equation [13], which describes the processes of population death rather well.

Hence, to optimize the multistage scenario of preclinical trials of $[^{25}Mg^{2+}]_4$PMC16 it is necessary to combine the system of in silico stroke equations presented above with the pharmacokinetic model of targeted delivery of $[^{25}Mg^{2+}]_4$PMC16 NPs to the ischemic penumbra zone.

10. Modeling the pharmacokinetics of fullerene-porphyrinic nano-cation exchangers carrying $^{25}Mg^{2+}$

The problems of modeling the pharmacokinetics of drugs have been studied extensively [14–16]. Such models are actively used in preclinical drug trials. Simultaneously, depending on the characteristics of the drugs under study, as well as the goals and objectives of such studies, one-chamber, two-chamber, three-chamber and four-chamber models are used.

The peculiarities of modeling the pharmacokinetics of fullerene-porphyrin nano-cation exchangers carrying $^{25}Mg^{2+}$ are that due to the spin effect of the $^{25}Mg^{2+}$ isotope, it hyperstimulates ATP synthesis, and due to the presence of the PMC16 "nanocontainer", it has the property of "targeted" delivery to the area of the brain damaged by hypoxia.

In general, the dynamic processes of pharmacokinetics are modeled using systems of ordinary differential equations of the form [13]:

$$\begin{cases} x = f(x(t), p) + \sum_{i=1}^{n} h(x(t), p) u_i(t) \\ y(t) = g(u(t), x(t), p) \end{cases} \tag{30}$$

Where x(t) – n-dimensional function of the state (in pharmacokinetics - drug dose), f(x(t), p) – a function that defines the structure of the model, p – s-dimensional vector of parameters characterizing the process under consideration (in pharmacokinetics, the rate of drug transfer between organs),

h – a function that defines the structure of the input data,

u(t) – function of the input data (in pharmacokinetics - the method of introducing the drug into the body),

y(t) – k-dimensional function of experimental data (in pharmacokinetics - drug concentration in blood and/or urine),

g – a function that links the model to the dimensions.

By supplementing the system of equations Eqs. (18)–(29) with the system Eq. (30), we obtain a mathematical model of the *In Silico* I level of selective accumulation of cation-exchange PMC16 nanoparticles in brain cells and tissues for preclinical studies of the neuroprotective potential of fullerene-porphyrin nano-cation exchangers carrying $^{25}Mg^{2+}$ in relation to the pathogenesis of ischemic stroke.

11. Discussion of how this model will be correlated to real experiments

With regard to the correlation of the model with the data from real experiments, it is necessary to take into account a number of important circumstances arising from the specifics of the task. Namely: first of all, it is necessary to align the experimental results with the ischemic stroke model. This subproblem includes the coordination of each of the above-mentioned physiological processes that accompany the pathogenesis of this disease, expressed with separate differential equations. Furthermore, based on the in silico of stroke, which is consistent with the empirics, the same coordination of the equations describing the pharmacokinetics of PMC 16 is required.

However, this work must be completed. In this sense, further improvement of the model is planned in two main areas:

1. Complication of hypotheses used for the modeling processes and expansion of the system of differential equations;

2. Adaptation to problem conditions of existing semi-empirical models describing non-Markov population dynamics (Gomperz model, Verhulst logistic model, population size model in a periodic environment, population model with a smaller critical number, etc.) [17].

All these scenarios require coordination of in silico with experimental data obtained from in vivo of laboratory animals, which presupposes the following studies:

1. Defining the parameters of biological processes subject to experimental control in vivo.

2. Defining the variables and coefficients of the differential equations of the mathematical model, which are to be agreed with the experimental data.

3. Adaptation and optimization of relevant semi-empirical models (equations) of population dynamics and approximation of their parameters to the tasks set.

4. Determination of optimal mathematical methods for approximation and interpolation of experimental data.

5. Structure development and database creation for in silico goals and objectives.

6. Literature search and extraction of experimental data obtained by third-party researchers (external data). Their assortment, classification, and entry into specialized databases.

7. Comparison of external and internal (obtained as part of the framework of our own research) experimental data.

8. Output of transfer functions. Clarification of the pharmacokinetic equations in relation to the different methods of drug administration.

9. Preparation of algorithms for computer models.

This mathematical simulation (modeling) approach is an appropriate *In Silico* tool designed to describe and predict the key pharmacokinetic patterns of the *in vivo* distribution and the brain tissue accumulation of Magnesium-25 carrying — releasing PMC16 nanoparticles.

This tool seems promising for meeting the specific expectations of pharmacologists searching for the optimal, efficient and economical ways of planning this distinctive pharmacophore preclinical research.

12. Conclusions and prospects

This work presents algorithms for *in silico* modeling of selective accumulation of cation-exchange PMC16 nanoparticles in cells and tissues of the brain for preclinical studies of the neuroprotective potential of fullerene-porphyrin nano-cation exchangers carrying $^{25}Mg^{2+}$ concerning the pathogenesis of ischemic stroke. Solving this problem is extremely important for the optimization of multistage scenarios of preclinical trials of $[^{25}Mg^{2+}]_4$PMC16 in experimental nanopharmacology of ischemic stroke. In the present study, these algorithms are in the spotlight.

As a result, we have obtained a relatively voluminous system of differential equations describing the pharmacokinetics of $[^{25}Mg^{2+}]_4$PMC16 in relation to the pathogenesis of ischemic stroke.

In systems in which several processes are implemented simultaneously, the difficulty of accurately solving the modeling problem increases in proportion to the number of processes taken into account. The search for a solution to such systems by analytical methods is rather difficult. In practice, one usually has to rely on approximate solutions or the use of numerical methods and computer simulation technologies. For this reason, we did not search for an analytical solution to the presented system of differential equations in the framework of this work.

As an alternative way aimed at simplifying the system of differential equations underlying *in silico*, one can use combinations of slightly modified systems of Gompertz equations and the non-Markov concept of population dynamics.

In our previous works [1–5, 18], these algorithms were partially presented and are not described in detail in this study but are our research's focus.

As seen from above, both Non-Markov population dynamics background and the Gompertz equation-based models were simultaneously applied here to harmonize a predicational pharmacokinetic validity and capabilities for the multivariant *In Silico* approach proposed for the Magnesium-25 releasing PMC16 nano-carriers as long as the latter are about to play a role of modulators of the brain hypoxia-related metabolic disorders.

Hereby, this is nothing more than an attempt to develop a simple and efficient computational tool applicable to optimize the decision-making process on exact steps and conditions of PMC16 engaging preclinical research strategy in the variable brain ischemia pharmacological studies.

Regarding the prospects for continuing work in this direction, it should be noted that at some point, as the algorithms become more complex, *in silico* formation without the use of artificial intelligence-based on computer neural networks will not be possible.

A further prospect of working on the *In Silico* project is to create conditions for bringing *In Silico* to the level of advanced smart technologies based on artificial intelligence neural networks.

Acknowledgements

Work was supported by grant of Ministry of Science and Higher Education of Russian Federation № 075-15-2020-792 (Unique identifier RF——190220X0031).

Author details

Valentin V. Fursov[1*], Ilia V. Fursov[2], Alexander A. Bukhvostov[1], Aleksander G. Majouga[3] and Dmitry A. Kuznetsov[1,4]

1 Pirogov Russian National Research Medical University, Moscow, Russia

2 Morozovskaya Children's City Clinical Hospital of the Department of Health of the City of Moscow, Moscow, Russia

3 D. Mendeleev University of Chemical Technology of Russia, Moscow, Russia

4 Lomonosov Moscow State University, Moscow, Russia

*Address all correspondence to: vfursov@mail.ru

References

[1] Sarkar, S., Rezayat, S.M., Buchachenko, A.L., Kuznetsov, D.A., Orlova, M.A., Yurovskaya, M.A., Trushkov, I.V. (2007) New water soluble porphylleren compounds. European Union Patent No. 07009882.7/EP07009882 (Reg.: Munich, Germany).

[2] Sarkar, S., Rezayat, S.M., Buchachenko, A.L., Kuznetsov, D.A., Orlova, M.A., Yurovskaya, M.A., Trushkov, I.V. (2007) Use of a magnesium isotope for treating hypoxia and a medicament comprising the same. European Union Patent No. 07009881.9/EP07009881 (Reg.: Munich, Germany).

[3] Buchachenko Anatoly L., Bukhvostov Alexander A., Ermakov Kirill V., Kuznetsov Dmitry A. 2020. A specific role of magnetic isotopes in biological and ecological systems. Physics and biophysics beyond. Progress in Biophysics and Molecular Biology 155 (2020) 1-19

[4] Stovbun, S.V., Vedenkin, A.S., Bukhvostov, A.A., Koroleva, L.S., Silnikov, V.N., Kuznetsov, D. A. L, 2020. D-Polydeoxyribonucleotides to provide an essential inhibitory effect on DNA polymerase β of human myeloid leukemia HL60 cells. Biochemistry and Biophysics Reports 24 (2020) 100835

[5] A. L. Buchachenko. Magneto-Biology and Medicine. Nova Biomedical Publ.: New York, 2015.

[6] M. Siccardi and A. Owen. Towards a computational prediction of nanoparticle pharmakokinetics and distribution. J. In Silico & In Vitro Pharmacol., 2(1):8–11, 2016.

[7] J. J. Augsburger, C. M. L. Chow, V. Dyer and M. F. Roussel. Translating science into survival. In: St. Jude's Children's Research Hospital Report (Cajjar, A. & Pappo, A., Eds.); St. Judes CRH Publ.: Memphis, TN — Cincinnati, OH:6–55, 2016.

[8] I. Bozic and M. A. Nowak. Resisting resistance. Ann. Rev. Cancer Biol., 1(1): 203–221, 2017.

[9] Gusev E.I.,Skvorcova V.I. Ishemiya golovnogo mozga. – M. : Medicina, 2001. – 328 s.

[10] J. Puyal, V. Ginet, P. G. H. Clarke. Multiple interacting cell death mechanisms in the mediation of excitotoxicity and ischemic brain damage: a challenge for neuroprotection. Prog. Neurobiol. 2013. Vol. 105. P. 24-48.

[11] Di Russo C. A mathematical model of inflammation during ischemic stroke / C. Di Russo et al. // ESAIM. – EDP Sciences. – 2010. – V. 30. – P. 15–33.

[12] N. D. Plotnikov, Ch. A. Cgoev, O. F. Voropaeva Matematicheskoe modelirovanie processov gibeli kletok v zhivom organizme. – Novosibirsk, 2017.

[13] I. D. Bassukas. Comparative Gompertzian analysis of alterations of tumor growth patterns. Cancer Res., 54 (16):4385–4392, 1994.

[14] A. V. Matveev Modelirovanie kinetiki radiofarmpreparatov s izotopami joda v zadachah yadernoj mediciny//Komp'yuternye issledovaniya i modelirovanie. – 2020. – T. 12. – № 4. – S. 883–905

[15] Kabanihin S.I., Voronov D.A., Grodz' A.A., Krivorot'ko O.I. Identificiruemost' matematicheskih modelej medicinskoj biologii. Vavilovskij zhurnal genetiki i selekcii. 2015;19(6):738-744. DOI 10.18699/VJ15.097-744

[16] V.F. Antonov i dr. – Biofizika. - M.: Vlados, 2000.

[17] S. V. Sokolov Modeli dinamiki populyacij: ucheb. posobie. SPb.: Izd-vo SPbGETU «LETI», 2018.

[18] Johansen, R.J., Bukhvostov, A.A., Ermakov, K.V., Kuznetsov, D.A. 2018. Towards a computational prediction for the tumor selective accumulation of paramagnetic nanoparticles in retinoblastoma cells. BULLETIN OF RSMU 6, 2018